THE WHOLE MAN
PROJECT

THE WHOLE MAN
PROJECT
THE MILITARY ATHLETE'S
PERFORMANCE MANUAL

JERAMIAH SOLVEN

ISBN: 978-1-961781-93-1

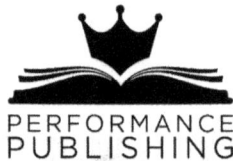

PERFORMANCE
PUBLISHING

To my family, the men I have served with, and the fallen.
"Arete"

CONTENTS

SECTION 1: THE MIND

WHY THE WHOLE MAN PROJECT?

W hy should you read this book or give this program a chance? It is because this book will give you a competitive edge in anything you do. It is a training manual for your body and mind. It includes actionable steps to transform the way you think and perform — steps that will push you to better yourself physically and mentally. It is the book I wish I had 15 years ago to propel myself to a higher level.

This program started out as a way for me to figure out one of the most difficult ways to train; to find a way to get stronger and faster, concurrently. Over time, it evolved into something much bigger. It became a model to train my body, mind, and soul — a vehicle to achieve a peak level of performance and growth. Over the last 16 years, I have shared these tools piece-by-piece, and consistently received overwhelmingly positive feedback. Success is an inside job; therefore, your results are completely dependent on your level of commitment and application. How you use the information between these covers is up to you. For those of you who are open to the concept that success is a mindset, this book is for you.

This is my attempt to store a copy of what I have learned about personal growth and fitness and to share the information with friends, family, and strangers to whom I am so deeply committed. I am excited to share what I have learned, and I am even more excited for your internal and external growth. I hope you enjoy.

APPRECIATION

Thank you to my parents Linda and Rick, for their constant encouragement and teaching me to never quit. To my wife Charyce, thank you for your unconditional love and support. Lastly, to all of my friends who have contributed to this book and my growth - without you there is no me.

ABOUT THE AUTHOR

This program was written by Jeramiah Andrew Solven. He holds a Bachelor of Science in Kinesiology with a concentration in Exercise Science and Clinical Health. He was an Army Infantry Officer and Ranger and has over 16 years of experience in physical training programming. He began writing fitness programs in high school for his friends at age 15 and then went on to earn his Personal Training Certification through the International Sports and Science Association (ISSA). He attained his undergraduate degree at California Polytechnic University, Pomona, and has a passion for training strength and endurance concurrently. Jeramiah has trained over 200 military athletes in his career, and his program was adopted by over 100 Military Officers in 2017. He has consistently increased the fitness level of every organization of which he has been a member. As a result of this 12-week program, his Maneuver Captain Career Course Seminar of 21 Combat Arms Officers attained the highest seminar average for the Army Physical Fitness Test and the 12-Mile Ruck March. Jeramiah's 12-week program is the cornerstone of "The Whole Man Project," which was designed to train the body and mind together to achieve physical peaks and mental growth.

If you want to learn more about Jeramiah, follow him on Instagram @jeramiahsolven or email him at info@jeramiahsolven.com.

MY STORY

I t is a bit difficult for me to write about myself; however, getting to know the author of a book is important. I find it makes the book more relatable. Knowing about the author helps me visualize what the author is conveying and helps me create an imaginary relationship with them. That imaginary relationship increases retention and makes the book more enjoyable for me. As an author, I would like you to get to know me so that you can get the most out of this book.

My name is Jeramiah Andrew Solven. I was raised in a town of fewer than 300 people in Northern California and spent my youth hunting and playing with my three brothers. I was undersized as a kid and discovered weight training as a method of combating my insecurities.

For some context, during my freshman year of high school I was 5'1 and 98 lbs. At 14, I joined the high school wrestling team and did everything within my power to become the best wrestler possible. I went to training camps, joined off-season teams, and turned wrestling into what could be considered a year-round sport. As time progressed, my dream was to compete at the highest levels and to become a champion. Along the way, I became infatuated with weight training as a method of improving my capabilities. I began writing my own workout programs, and by 15 I started doing the same for my friends and classmates. I had dreams of becoming a personal trainer and wrestling my way through college.

As the years progressed, I got better and better at wrestling, and during my senior year of high school I trained to be a state place winner. That was one of the most intense and demanding years of my life. I trained two to three times a day and obsessed over winning and reaching my potential. During the last tournament of the season, I competed in a "true second" match. In previous years, the winner of the "true second match" would go on to compete at the State Championship. I competed in the toughest match of my high school career and went into overtime with my opponent. With seconds left on the clock, I won the match.

The win was, however, bittersweet. After I was announced the winner, my coach came to me ecstatic, but I sensed sadness as he approached. He told me true second winners were not allowed to go to state that year.

Looking back at my life as I write this, that moment impacted me more than I ever thought possible. In my mind, I had failed at becoming the elite wrestler I dreamed of. I began to talk myself out of all of my goals. I talked myself out of becoming a personal trainer after listening to the advice of people close to me. Those people criticized that I should "get a real job," so I listened and got one at a local hardware store. I gave up on my dreams and decided to follow what was "normal."

Following high school, I attended a community college. Feeling empty and lost, I dropped out after two months. I made the decision to enlist in the Army and pursue a job that "made sense." I enlisted in 2005 as an engineer. I deployed to Iraq in 2006, and for 15 months I reflected on the life I had made. I became angry and disappointed with the way I had given up on my interests.

Then in 2007, a trigger went off in my head. I got fed up with my circumstances and became convicted about pursuing my passions. I cannot describe how, but I became so dissatisfied with my life I could not stand living another day in it. I made the decision to stop living for everyone else and start living for myself.

I enjoyed some aspects of being in the Army, but I did not enjoy the job I was in. I told myself I wanted to make a difference and do something more challenging. I chose to go back to school, to finish what I had started and learn about the human body. I earned a B.S. in Kinesiology, Exercise Science through the Army's Green to Gold Scholarship Program. I then attained a personal training certification from the International Sports and Science Association (ISSA).

Following college, I completed the Infantry Basic Officer Leader Course (IBOLC) and earned my commission as an Infantry Officer. I have attended numerous military courses to include the U.S. Army Ranger School. It was during the time I went to Ranger School that "The Whole Man Concept" was born. I had started accumulating small victories across my military career and my confidence was returning. The Whole Man Concept became a model for determining what I wanted out of life. It evolved into a tool for self-reflection and a catalyst for this program: The Whole Man Project.

I have used The Whole Man Concept to go forth and serve within the 75th Ranger Regiment and manifest my deepest desires. However, what is important to note is that the Whole Man model pushed me beyond what I thought was possible. Using this model, I was able to achieve intense physical accomplishments that I otherwise would not have had the confidence to attempt.

One of the first physical feats that the Whole Man model propelled me to do was transform my endurance. I went from routinely only running less than five miles to competing in the Army's Best Ranger Competition (BRC). BRC was my first real endurance event. I traveled over 50 miles on foot in approximately 20 hours, with and without a ~50lb rucksack.

Another result of the Whole Man model was that it enabled me to run my first marathon, which I ended up doing on a treadmill. Yes, the full 26.2 miles.

Why a treadmill? Well, The Whole Man Concept helped me generate a goal of running a marathon. During that time, I was deployed, and because of a suicide bomber attack, running outside was not authorized. I used three different treadmills to "mix it up" and completed the marathon after work one day while deployed. The guys I served with came in and laughed at me for spending so much time on a treadmill. When they asked why I was running a marathon on a treadmill, I told them it was because I had said I was going to. I could not help but laugh to myself, knowing the burning desire I had to uphold my goal. The Whole Man Concept sparked something in me that I could not deny. It helped me create purpose and direction in my life and scale unprecedented heights.

The Whole Man Concept is the reason I attained my fastest 12-mile ruck time of 1 hour and 57 minutes. I have used it to improve my eating habits. I have used it to test many trending diets so I could speak intelligently of their processes and applications afterward.

The Whole Man Concept is the method I used to manifest my dream and serve with some of the military's top members in special operations. I never imagined I would go from being a small-town kid to fighting alongside heroes in armed combat. The Whole Man Concept is what I have used to completely transform my life in numerous domains.

Through it all, what I am most proud of is that I can share this method with you.

INTRODUCTION

"Life is long if you know how to use it."
~Seneca

What you do in one area of your life, you do in all. Therefore, it is my belief that you should use fitness to practice the habits necessary to reach the greatest version of your ideal self. Throughout the program, you will attack each workout to reconstruct your belief system, develop resiliency, and harden the body, mind, and soul. The program is designed to develop the athlete physically and mentally over the course of 12 weeks. You will start unlocking your potential by training your mind, and then transition to training the body. Throughout the book, I will give you tools to use to tend to your soul and subconscious.

When you get to the fitness section of the book, you will notice every week has a lesson. The lessons will be pulled from the mental training in the beginning of this book. It will give you the opportunity you will need to actively rehearse the lessons and incorporate them into your life through fitness. You will learn how to generate momentum in your day through habits and routines. It will show you how to achieve a peak state by changing your mind and behaviors.

It is through mindset shifts that you begin to create radically different results.

A clear example of the way mindset can affect outcome is outlined by the experiences of two Noncommissioned Officers (NCOs) with whom I had the pleasure of serving. These two NCOs could have been twins. They were war heroes, intellectuals, and highly ambitious. Both served in special operations and had similarities; however, they differed in mindset.

These two individuals attended a Noncommissioned Officer Enlisted School, and both soldiers believed the course was an inconvenience and below their level of expertise. I knew the school would be hard-pressed to challenge the two of them, and sympathized that they were required to attend.

Two stellar NCOs (let's name them Alpha and Bravo) departed for the school, yet came back with completely contrasting results. NCO Alpha came back as an honor graduate, while NCO Bravo barely passed. I was baffled at the outcome. Both were high performers, competitors, and winners, so why did they yield such different results?

When I asked them about their individual experiences, NCO Bravo told me he did not want to be there, and he did not care about doing well. In contrast, NCO Alpha informed me that he also hated every second he was there, BUT he told himself he had to get the most out of it and learn SOMETHING. Every day, NCO Alpha applied himself. It was not about getting a good grade; it was about doing the best he could while representing his organization to the highest standard. His performance was a direct reflection of his character.

As you see by the example, how we communicate to ourselves about the obstacles ahead of us determines the result. The ability to effectively control our thoughts and mind can be the difference between barely passing life and winning it. To achieve a higher level of performance, start with the mind. In order to get what we want out of life, we have to become masters of our minds, and not the servants of our thoughts.

Everyone has moments in life where the fruits of their labor have been either bolstered or hindered by their mindset. I know I have. In order to break through mindset barriers, holding all activities to the same standard will propel you to a higher level of performance. What you do in one area of your life, you do in all. Using that mindset, I have utilized fitness as a focal point to teach myself lessons, grow, and become a better version of myself each day. Changing my mindset has changed my life more than I ever thought possible.

Next, I am going to share with you The Whole Man Concept, which is the cornerstone of The Whole Man Project. I created The Whole Man Concept to establish purpose in my life, while simultaneously pushing myself to a higher level. The Whole Man Concept allows you to define what balance and fulfillment look like in your life. The project is a great tool that allows you to slow down your fast-paced life, take a look at the big picture, and determine what areas of your life have been neglected. Understanding what balance looks like can help us align our days and life with our unique visions of success. Success within The Whole Man Concept is relative to the individual; there is no right answer, only *your* answer.

The first step of any journey is awareness of the path ahead. After awareness, the goal is gathering the tools — or as I like to say the "golden nuggets" — for growth. Both people and books have these nuggets, in my opinion. I call them nuggets because gathering tools for personal growth is a bit like panning for gold (yes, I have done some prospecting in my day).

You sit in a creek bed, pan in hand; you sieve through water and sand to find one small piece of gold that will change your life. It takes time and patience, but the moment you think you have found something, your whole perspective changes and you become something just a little bit different, just a little bit better than you were before. Like panning for gold, prospecting for information in books offers a similar reward.

Nuggets generate inflection points. An inflection point is a point in your path where you have two choices: you can stay on your current trajectory or give growth a chance and explore unknown territory. Sometimes it takes reading an entire book to find the one nugget you are going to use, but at the end, if that nugget is life-changing, it is all worth it.

My hope is that you find at least one nugget in this book, something that changes your perspective and pushes you to become a better version of yourself. Even if you find nothing, there are still some killer workouts for you to get after.

HOW TO USE THIS BOOK

As you begin reading, you will notice a military undertone as a recurring theme. I chose to do that intentionally; there are a myriad of parallels between daily life and the military, specifically combat. I believe LIFE is combat. Each day we step into a different battle; it is up to us to prepare for it, plan for it, and ultimately DOMINATE it. Some days we feel inspired, other days we do not. Regardless of our level of inspiration, life causes us to shed blood, struggle, and fight. In the end, we all want the same thing: to WIN.

Think of this book as a field manual for the combat you face in your own life. It will keep you focused on your "objective" and provide you with actionable tools to adjust your routines and behaviors. I encourage you to highlight parts that stand out to you and come back to them after you finish for further growth and fine-tuning. The model I've created supports a continued process for personal growth, and more importantly, it's tailored to the individual.

The Whole Man Project is designed to train the body, the mind, and the soul. I have split it into two sections: the first section covers the mind, and the second encompasses the body. Throughout both sections, we will tend to the soul.

In the first section, "The Mind," I will give you the tools I have used to invoke SUSTAINABLE growth in my life. I am naturally a habitual person, as are most humans. The first section will teach you how to take control of your habits and develop new routines. Additionally, the first section will introduce the power of specificity and walk you through a goal-setting strategy. My intention is to teach you how to manage yourself, then give you tools to develop laser-sharp focus.

The second section, "The Body," contains a structured workout routine that applies the concepts learned from "The Mind." Combining the mindset techniques and workout program will make you an unstoppable force. Simply put, this book was written for individuals who are looking for an edge. The information throughout will give you the tools you need to separate yourself from your peers and win.

The workouts alone are tailored for intermediate athletes — individuals who played a sport in high school and currently accumulate at least five to 10 miles of running a week. Additionally, the workout program was built for combat arms service members who are familiar with rucking. The program was tailored to fit the needs of high-level athletes who want to set new personal records in the five-mile run and 12-mile ruck while improving their strength. If the workout is too intense for you, you can always modify your runs (by half for beginners) and lifts (to suit your current fitness level). Bottom line: make it manageable for yourself, prevent injuries, and use fitness to build the foundation for your personal growth.

Reference the workout program at the end of the book. It is 12 weeks long and you will notice at week nine the program becomes less prescriptive with your self-study. I have chosen to write the program in a way that allows you to learn as you go and become self-sufficient by the end. I have designed the book with a "Crawl, Walk, Run" methodology.

Reading the material of the book is the Crawl Phase. You will study and gather the information necessary to execute the 12-week workout plan. In the Walk Phase, you will execute the workouts and be assigned specific study material to further your knowledge. In the Run Phase, you will have all the tools necessary to execute the workout program and be provided flexibility in your self-study and become self-sustaining.

By this point, you will have instilled the habits and routines necessary for continued growth. After understanding the daily battle rhythm, you will be able to further fine-tune your goals and continue to advance on your own. At the end of the book, I will walk you through steps to create your own workout routine by taking you through a concept I use to write mine. Now that you know how to use this book, we are going to step into the first section and unlock your weakest link: your mind.

SECTION ONE
THE MIND

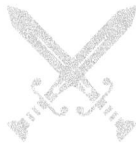

AWARENESS

"Vague beginnings cause chaotic endings."
~ Anonymous

The first step to improving yourself is acknowledging you need to change. In order to change, we have to accept the idea that we are capable of more than we are currently giving.

We cannot increase our capacity until we realize our potential. We have to accept there is more "out there" than we are currently living and begin looking for ways to expand our context. Think of this concept like two goldfish raised in a bowl. Both fish are swimming around, and one goldfish is trying to convince the other that there is more to life than the bowl in which they live. The stubborn goldfish is content swimming in circles, not amounting to anything more, while the other craves something outside the bowl but does not know what exists. The goldfish that refuses to accept that there is more to life fails to acknowledge its level of incompetence.

There are four stages for developing a skill or learning new information, namely unconscious incompetence, conscious incompetence, conscious competence, and unconscious competence. I would like to focus your attention on the first stage: unconscious incompetence.

In this first stage, an individual lacks awareness of his/her circumstances. A person who joins the military and has never fired a weapon before can make their best guess as to how to shoot, but will fail to get better at shooting if they ignore the fact they shoot poorly. They will only get better if they consciously become aware they lack the skills necessary to shoot well.

Creating awareness moves us from stage one to stage two: conscious incompetence. It is the stage in learning where you acknowledge your shortcomings at the task at hand. It is simply the point during skill development where you know you need to work on the skill to get better.

The third stage, conscious competence, is when you are doing something right, but you have to focus on doing it the right way. In our shooting example, it means learning the fundamentals of marksmanship and focusing on them before every trigger squeeze. As your skills increase, the action becomes reflexive and you move into the fourth stage, unconscious competence. In this stage you are on autopilot and you do not have to focus deeply to get the desired result. The action becomes reflexive, and you can unconsciously fire your weapon with stunning accuracy. The key to moving up the "competence ladder" is to expand what we know. Donald Rumsfeld said, "We do not know what we do not know";

therefore, I am going to share with you one tool I use to decrease "what I do not know" and increase my awareness.

In order to increase my awareness, I focus on increasing my CONTEXT. I use the word context deliberately. Robert Kiyosaki is a real estate professional, financial expert, and author. He claims in order to become an expert in something we have to INCREASE CONTEXT so that we can add more CONTENT. If you think of a glass of water, the context is the glass and the content is the water. We are limited regarding how much water we can fit in the glass by the size of the glass, or by what is known as the context. If we want to put more content in our glass, then we need a bigger glass; we need to understand that there are bigger glasses out there and it is up to us to discover them.

Fortunately, by reading this book, you are already increasing your awareness. Picking up this book separates you from everyone who hasn't. The more you expose yourself to, the broader your context.

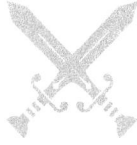

ONE PERCENT BETTER

"The journey of a thousand miles begins with a single step."
~ Lao Tzu

The next step in this program is to accept the challenge of becoming 1% better every day. Rapid growth in technology has created a culture that glorifies instant gratification and lack of patience. While I value impatience as a strength because it generates urgency, I also think being patient and slowly, progressively stacking wins is extremely powerful.

Instead of trying to become 100% better overnight, the focus of this program is to become 1% better each day. If you dedicate yourself to becoming 1% better every day, in 100 days you become 100% better. Refrain from focusing on the end state, and capitalize on the habit of making incremental improvements. Trying to get 1% better each day is not only achievable; it is sustainable. Making too big a leap and failing every day is discouraging and can leave us thinking that the results we want are impossible. Reverse engineering the outcome we desire and attempting to gain "inches, not miles" will build your confidence and create massive amounts of momentum.

In Jim Collins' book *Good to Great*, he studied 28 successful companies and how they made the climb to "greatness." He realized the one common trait in each of the companies was the ability to take complex information and make it simple, effectively "mak[ing] the problem smaller." I like to use reading as an example. Many people claim to want to read more, and frankly, I used to be the same. I began by "mak[ing] the problem smaller." I dedicated each day to completing at least one sentence. If I did not have the time to read one sentence, I lost the entire day. As I stacked wins each day, I increased the amount I read. As a result I went from NEVER reading a full book in 10 years to reading 42 books in 52 weeks. I missed my goal because I prioritized military training and went to the National Training Center in Fort Irwin. However, at the end of the year, I was still impressed with how much I had learned. Recently, my most impressive "win" was reading a 250- to 300-page book in two hours while waiting for a flight at the airport.

If you do not have time for a full sentence, make the goal a word a day. Start to scale your efforts and when you reach consistent failure, pull back and continue to focus on the routine. Think about something you have been meaning to do, and figure out a way to do just a little bit of it each day. Reward yourself after completion to reinforce the new behavior. I like to reward myself with some type of activity that makes me laugh. It could be a phone call, an evening out with friends, or a movie. Remember to reward yourself with a positive habit, not a destructive one.

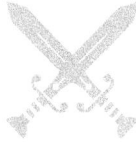

A BATTLE DRILL
FOR CHANGE

*"Insanity is doing the same thing over and
over, but expecting a different result."*
~ Albert Einstein

O nce you are aware that you can personally improve
and make a personal conviction to become 1% better each and every day, the next step is to develop
a system for change. The system I created mirrors an Army
Battle Drill.

In the Army, a battle drill is an action rapidly executed
without applying a deliberate decision-making process. Battle
drills allow for quick reaction with limited thinking. They
are executed in high-stress environments in order to close
with and destroy the enemy, and that is precisely what we
are trying to do with our old self. You cannot change without
an effective system any more than a squad can execute Battle
Drill 1A (Squad Attack) without practicing it first.

I have four steps that I execute like a battle drill to create change. I have used these steps in numerous areas of my life to include my personal finances. When I decided I wanted to become wealthy, I used them to completely reverse my finances and put myself into a climbing progression toward wealth. I have even used these steps in fitness.

When I wanted to get big and increase my weight, I used these steps to break through my existing plateau. I used them to go from weighing 170 lbs. to 200 lbs. in muscle mass over the course of six months. I call on them to completely destroy what I have done in the past and achieve new results. Most people are convinced they can achieve a different outcome and still repeat their past behaviors. Through experience, I completely disagree. These are the kind of people who look the same every year in the gym and cannot understand why. I am guilty of the same behavior and that is why I created this "Battle Drill for Change" to keep myself evolving. Any time you want to change an area in your life, reference it to get yourself producing different results.

The Battle Drill for Change is:

1.   Become aware.
2.   Think like an inventor.
3.   Create the routine.
4.   Practice the opposite.

I will expand on the four-step "Battle Drill for Change" in the paragraphs that follow.

Step #1 – Become aware.

In a previous chapter, we discussed awareness in depth. We also discussed "what got you here won't get you there." Step one of the Battle Drill for Change nests within that belief. We will remain the same unless we take the first step and acknowledge that we need to change. In professional sports, when an athlete cannot find a way to break a personal record, they become aware they need to do something different and change their approach.

Roger Bannister is a prime example of an athlete whose first step toward becoming a champion was awareness. In 1952, Roger competed in the 1500m race at the Olympics. But much to his disappointment, he failed to medal. After recovering mentally from the loss and almost quitting racing, Roger made the decision to continue to compete but to do things differently. He became aware he wanted to break the world record four-minute mile.

He intensified his training and increased his speed work. Then on May 6th 1954 Roger Bannister broke the world record and accomplished what others deemed impossible. He finished the one-mile race in 3:59.4 and changed history.

Becoming aware is the first step of the Battle Drill for Change because it is the most important. Increase your awareness by increasing your context and move on to step two for continued change.

Step #2 – Think like an inventor.

Inventors are eager to get through what does not work so that they can get to what does work. They welcome failed attempts to learn through their mistakes and make progress.

It took Thomas Edison 10,000 attempts to create the light bulb. When interviewed he said, "I did not fail 10,000 times, I just found 10,000 ways that did not work."

The second step in the battle drill is to approach the area in your life you want to change like an inventor. Adopt the mindset of experimenting; the "invention" you are trying to create is success. I have used the Battle Drill for Change in my workouts. When I notice I have reached a plateau and become aware I need to do things differently, I approach all of my workouts with an inventing mindset. I want to create change, and I want to change my physical ability. Therefore, I will review my past workouts and ask the questions: "What worked and what did not work?" The answer reveals what I should do more of and less of. If doing the traditional workout routine of three to four sets for 10-12 repetitions isn't working, it is time to do something different. It is time to experiment with different rep ranges, exercises, and lifting techniques.

A lot of people do not realize that small alterations can make drastic changes. Changing your spacing in a lift is a great example of making a small change to gain significant results. If I normally do wide squats, I will take a narrow stance. Instead of putting my effort into the concentric portion of the lift, I will focus my effort on the eccentric. I will make small changes and test their effectiveness by assessing my fatigue and soreness. Through trial and error, you will discover what works best for you.

You will notice when you start to approach one area of your life like an inventor, you will start applying it to others. I have had several occasions where I have started testing things in my workouts and then began noticing the other things in my life that were and were not working. Keep track of your research in a notebook, annotate it, and learn from your trials. Once you discover what does work, it is time to double down your efforts. Again, this concept does not just apply to fitness. Think of the results you would achieve in your relationships if you doubled down, and in your finances if you adopted the same approach. If it is working just a little bit, do more of it and you will get more.

Step #3 – Create the routine.

Once you discover what works, it is time to construct a new routine around your success. In step two, we used reaching a physical plateau as an example of something we wanted to change. In step three, it is time to create the routine to map out your workouts for the week. After you have identified the techniques and/or exercises that are shocking your body (causing you to be sore/fatigued), draft up a plan to do more of them. Plug those new methods into your training plan and double down on your efforts. For example, if you're trying to develop your pectoral muscles and while "inventing" you discover alternate dumbbell presses are breaking down the muscle fibers and causing soreness, plan to do them every Monday. Double down on your efforts by implementing alternate dumbbell presses into multiple exercises — incline, decline, and flat elevations.

Creating a new routine means becoming deliberate architects of what we want to achieve. I am constantly using fitness as the focus point throughout this book because like I said at the beginning, "what you do in one area of your life you do in all." If you can apply the Battle Drill for Change to fitness, then you can apply it to anything and achieve profound results.

I have used the Battle Drill for Change to become spiritually balanced. When I was younger, I developed a distaste for religion, but as the years progressed, it was something I wanted to have in my life. I used The Whole Man Concept (which we will talk about later) to identify and improve that area of my life. I wanted to find a way to increase my faith and partnership with my Higher Power. I already knew what did not work (church), so after becoming aware I wanted to increase my faith, I started to think like an inventor and began experimenting. I found that meditation and gratitude worked. I doubled down on my efforts and created a routine that allowed me time to practice meditation and gratitude daily. My perspective toward the world and attitude completely shifted in a positive way.

Step three of the Battle Drill for Change helped me create a daily routine to achieve my spiritual goal.

When executing the Battle Drill for Change, I prefer to make massive routine changes, not small adjustments. Massive changes shock your body and put it into a state of unfamiliarity. There is no time for the mind to convince you to fall back on the old routines because it is occupied with figuring out how to survive with the new ones. Have you ever seen somebody lose an incredible amount of weight when they move to a new environment, only to gain it all back when they fall back into their old routine? They rebound because they put themselves too close to their old routines and they subconsciously gravitate toward their old behaviors.

A new routine should keep you from falling back into old behaviors. One tool I use to keep the new routine fresh in my mind is to approach everything I do with the mindset that I am going to do everything differently than I used to. I like to keep the idea that I am working on change by executing the next step of the Battle Drill, "Practice the Opposite."

Step #4 – Practice the opposite.

In order to keep your mind in a state of change, try making a habit of "practicing the opposite." Practicing the opposite means approaching all of the daily activities differently. By doing so, the idea of change is reinforced. From the moment you wake up, take any routine habit you have, and do the opposite action of what you are used to. Treat small and large habits the same.

Start by changing the smallest details of your day. For instance, if you normally open the door with your right hand, try opening it with your left. Instead of your usual trek to work, try a more scenic route. Same parking area at the grocery store? Park on the opposite side. Making small changes throughout your day compounds the overall message of change to your inner self. You will be sending subconscious messages to yourself that tell your body to pull out of its routines and behaviors and start building new ones. Practicing doing things differently than you are used to helps keep the idea of change in the forefront of your mind. Additionally, you will notice you will start to be more and more aware of how much control you have over changing anything you want.

I cannot count the number of people I interact with on day-to-day basis who feel change is outside of their control.

I often hear them say: "I wish I could eat healthy... I wish I could look the way that guy does." The truth is, they just have not developed a system for change that gives them the confidence they can control those outcomes. All it takes to change is to create thoughts that make you feel like you can. And creating those thoughts starts with paying attention to what you think about.

The brain has a system called the Reticular Activating System (RAS). To put it simply, the RAS is responsible for filtering in the information you are looking for and keeping out what you are not. In this step of the Battle Drill, practicing the opposite keeps the RAS looking for new ways to approach activities. Your RAS will look for things that are different and you will become more aware of things that could help you. Have you ever bought a new truck and the next thing you know there are five of the same truck in your neighborhood? That is the RAS taking control. Activating your RAS with the idea that you are looking for change will help create a mind that pulls you out of your old behaviors and into new ones.

I am always looking for ways to change and get better, and the Battle Drill for Change is the system I have created to help me with it. I have used this step to break past plateaus in the gym. This battle drill has helped me change it up in the gym to get out of my past behaviors and target my muscles differently.

The steps I have just laid out are a tool to create change in your life. Adopt my system if you would like, but more importantly, create a system that works for you.

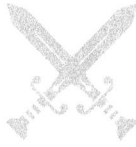

MANAGING ONESELF
AND ONE'S DECISIONS

*"The world is not a crazy enough of a place to
reward a bunch of undeserving people."*
~ Charlie Munger.

The goal of this first section — "The Mind" — is to give you tools (mindset techniques, routines, and rituals) to invoke sustainable growth into your life. This section is titled "The Mind" because we are training the way we think. The Mind section is designed to rebuild the way you approach life so that you can achieve more. Through this process you have developed **A**wareness you can do more, you have committed to becoming 1% **B**etter each day, and you have learned a method to **C**hange your current trajectory and break through plateaus. Up to this point if you have implemented the tools provided, you have completely destroyed your old self and you are asking "What next?" The next step toward growth is developing the ability to make the best decisions possible to increase your physical and mental performance.

Decisions are the steppingstone toward what we deserve. If we make poor decisions, we deserve poor results. If we work out hard but decide to eat cake at every meal, we still deserve to be fat. Over the last 10 years, I have studied the people around me who cannot figure out how to deserve more. These are the type of people who never seem to meet their goals. I often see them struggle with understanding why they cannot achieve more. But the reason is simple: they have never earned it.

To give you an example, the Army's Physical Fitness Test is a requirement for all soldiers regardless of rank. It is comprised of a timed two-mile run, timed push-ups, and timed sit-ups. Soldiers often want to score high on the APFT but gripe and complain about their scores when they are low. However, the reason they did not score as high as they wanted is because they did not put in the work to get there. Anybody who wants to increase what they deserve has to take responsibility for their outcome and learn to make decisions that entitle them to more.

Part of training your mind is developing the ability to control the various factors that influence your decision making. I have determined there are three key factors that influence decision making and thus influence what we deserve. These factors are: our social environment, our physiology (genetics), and our emotions. Specifically, the people around us, our genetic predisposition, and how we feel all influence how we plan, prepare, act, and succeed.

I have learned that to maximize our growth in any facet of life, we have to be able to control each of these three factors so that they serve us. Allow me to break down the three influencers of how we make decisions and give you specific actions to manipulate each of them.

The three influencers of how we make decisions are:

1. Social Environment
2. Genetics
3. Emotions

1.) Social Environment

The first factor that influences how we make decisions is our social environment. The law of averages states "The final product of any situation will be the average of all possible conclusions." Congruently, speaker and entrepreneur Jim Rohn said: "You are the average of the five people you spend the most time with." If you compare yourself to those around you, it is likely that there is only a 20% difference between you and those in your social circle.

Whether you compare finances, credit score, quality of life, or even political affiliation, humans naturally gravitate toward like-minded individuals. We crave becoming members of "the tribe." By becoming members of the tribe, we are rewarded with the feeling of acceptance and removed from feeling like an outcast. As we integrate into our social environments, we begin to adopt the thoughts and beliefs of those around us. Slowly, we begin to resemble and act as those around us.

Understanding that our social environment shapes us, it is important that we do not allow it to pull us down. The Crab Theory is a related concept of the way our environment can pull us toward an undesirable outcome. When you fill a bucket halfway with crabs, the crabs on the bottom will prevent any crab from trying to escape. They will grab the legs of the crabs that crawl above them. Unwittingly, they will pull the higher crab back into the bucket in an attempt to gain freedom for themselves. Humans mirror this behavior. Have you ever tried to do something unusual that your parents or friends thought was abnormal? They naturally try to convince you not to act on the change. Little do they know, they are acting in line with crab mentality.

Just as our social environment can bring us down, it can bring us up and help us reach a new level of success. I like to think of this concept in terms of real estate. If you buy the smallest home in a neighborhood with mansions, the mansions bring up the small home's value. Likewise, on sports teams and even in the military, the more "valuable" players hold each other accountable for poor performance. If you are performing below the standard, the team will put pressure on you to do better. You can watch just about any sports game and see the players encourage each other so the team performs better. They actively help the distracted player regain his focus and the angry player calm down, all in an attempt to win the game.

Now that you are aware your environment shapes you, you can use it as a tool to increase your outcome. If you want to naturally increase your performance, find a better team and they will force it out of you.

How do you find a better team? First, let me tell you this is something that is in your complete control. Deciding where you spend your time is a choice. You will have to get past what you have done previously, but the good thing is that we have already developed the skills to change. If you draw a blank when trying to determine where to spend your time, just ask the questions "What type of person do I want to be around?" and "Where would they spend their time?" Let the answers drive where you go. If you repeat that process enough, you will eventually cross paths with the exact type of person/group you are looking for. You will be destined for a new social environment and destined for better decisions.

2.) Personality Traits

Personality traits are the second factor that influence how we make decisions. They are responsible for how we approach and process the world around us. At the subconscious level, we all make decisions that are inherent to us. We make them based on how we are genetically constructed. Personality traits are the reason outgoing people seek out being around people. They are the reason some people lie more than others, and they are the reason some people conform to peer pressure, and some do not.

In this section, I am going to teach you how to gain control over your personality traits so that you will become better at managing yourself. You will begin to understand how you unconsciously make decisions so that you have the awareness to adjust them as needed. I have two tools to help you assess and later modify your personality traits. By using these tools, you will be able to get an "under the hood" look at how your mind works, and will gain control of how you inherently make decisions.

The first tool is a book titled *The H-Factor of Personality: Why Some People Are Manipulative, Self-Entitled, Materialistic, and Exploitive—And Why It Matters for Everyone*. In this book, Doctors Kibeom Lee and Michael C. Ashton provide scientific evidence and analysis of six personality dimensions: Honesty-Humility, Emotionality, Extroversion, Agreeableness, Conscientiousness, and Openness to New Experience. The doctors analyze the pairing of Honesty with the other five traits. Reading this book will give you a better understanding of how each trait contributes to how a person makes decisions.

For example, in the book, Honesty and Agreeableness are presented as two of the six traits that make up the human personality. These traits contribute directly to our decision-making process. Have you ever met somebody who makes very honest decisions? They typically have a difficult time lying and they will almost always make honest decisions over dishonest ones. These are the type of people who have a hard time keeping secrets. They are likely to "spill the beans" before a big surprise. How about a person who makes decisions just to be agreeable? People with high levels of Agreeableness will say yes to things they do not necessarily want to just to appease people around them. Understanding the six personality dimensions will help you increase your self-awareness. It will help you identify which dimensions may be leading you into making poor decisions. Studying the six personality dimensions will help you begin to understand which traits are naturally guiding you on a day-to-day basis.

Now that you are aware of the personality traits that define you, you can gain control of them and design who you want to be. The second tool I recommend to supplement the book is an online quiz that measures your levels of Honesty-Humility, Emotionality, Extroversion, Agreeableness, Conscientiousness, and Openness. It is called the HEXACO personality trait quiz. You can find the quiz at http://hexaco. org/. It takes 15 minutes and will give you an assessment of where you fall on the spectrum of each dimension and its sub-dimensions.

For example, the Conscientiousness dimension has sub-categories of Diligence, Organization, and Discipline. Have you ever met a person who seems incapable of being neat? Well, part of that reason is that they have a low Organization trait as a sub-dimension of the Conscientiousness dimension. If a person wants to get better at becoming organized, they must practice improving the Conscientiousness/Organization traits they have. Luckily, all it takes to make lasting change is structured, routine practice.

Self-improvement is a constant life progression. In my pursuit of the next level of myself, I have used both of the previous tools to modify my personality traits and make better decisions. One of my weaknesses in the past was diligence. I used to get so task-focused that I would miss steps trying to get to the result. In the end, the decision to bypass details would yield a poor result. By understanding my Conscientiousness trait, I have been able to understand that I have average levels of diligence and not exceptional levels.

By acknowledging that shortcoming, I have been able to improve on it daily. Diligence played a significant role in writing this book. I knew before writing it that I would need help with being thorough. By understanding my personality traits, I created a plan to ensure this book was well written. I created a redundant system and had several people review it to compensate for any details I might have missed on my own. In summary, addressing my diligence helped me make decisions around creating a quality product.

Understanding your personality traits will give you the power to be able to make better decisions. Like I said at the beginning of this chapter, decisions are the steppingstones toward what we deserve. If I had never addressed my diligence, I would never deserved have to be an author. Now, use the two tools I have listed to start understanding how your traits affect you, and begin working on them to change what you deserve.

3.) Emotions

The final factor that influences our decisions is our emotions. Anger, excitement, fear, and other feelings all influence our trajectory in life. They can cause us to fear and talk ourselves out of applying for a prestigious school, or get us overly excited and cause us to impulsively make a purchase we later regret. Part of training the mind is gaining control of these emotions so they do not persuade you to do something you might regret later.

By learning to control your emotions, you will develop the ability to continuously make decisions that benefit you. As I mentioned in the beginning of this chapter, you get what you deserve in life. In order to deserve more, we have to make decisions that entitle us to more.

This final, third factor in this chapter, "Managing Oneself and One's Decisions," is about developing the ability to separate how you feel from how you act so that you make logical, beneficial decisions that serve you.

Over my military career, I have seen people respond to events with their emotions and change their trajectory for the worse. From my observations, allowing emotions to control how you act will backfire. In the early days of my commission as an Army officer, I once saw a superior officer make an emotional decision to berate a subordinate because he felt disrespected. He demonstrated no restraint and many others saw him lash out. As time passed, he continued to make similar decisions to publicly humiliate those under him. Other officers stopped respecting him, and eventually stopped working for him. He became completely ineffective in the workplace. Had he learned to control his emotions, he could have done well, and I would be telling a different story.

For those who cannot relate to my military example, getting out of bed in a timely manner is an emotional decision with which most can identify. Refraining from hitting the snooze button can be a difficult task when it is early in the morning and you are not fully awake. It can be emotionally tough getting up on the first alarm. Even though waking up quicker is a decision that will give you more time in the day, emotions can interrupt that progress. The feeling of exhaustion can cause you to hit the snooze button several times. By the time you know it, you have wasted 30 minutes of your morning, or worse, been late to work.

In contrast, people who can control their emotions prosper. I believe that one of the main reasons I was accepted into the 75th Ranger Regiment was that I did not allow my emotions to control my decision to apply. Like anyone trying to do something harder, I struggled with the emotions of doubt and fear. I told myself I was not good enough or smart enough before I even picked up an application. Applying to special operations was intimidating. I watched a number of my peers talk themselves out of applying because they doubted their abilities. To get past my self-doubt, I made the decision to listen to logic and not feeling. I refused to allow my emotions to be the deciding factor in whether I applied. Looking back on it, breaking through those limiting beliefs was one of the greatest things I have done. My time in the 75th Ranger Regiment was one of the happiest seasons in my life.

You might already be happy with the way you handle your emotions. Nonetheless, we can always do better. One way I try to tame my emotions is with the "The Five Second Rule." This rule allows me to strengthen the ability to listen to logic over emotions.

The Five Second Rule

"The Five Second Rule" is a concept created by author Mel Robbins to achieve your goals. Check out her book *The 5 Second Rule* for more information. To put it simply, the Five Second Rule is one tool that you can use to keep your emotions from preventing you from doing something that will benefit you. The conflict when you are faced with making a painful decision usually occurs between what you understand (your logic) and how you feel (your emotions). The snooze button example previously mentioned is a situation in which the idea of getting out of bed quickly is beneficial but feels painful. Lying in bed contemplating when to get up burns time — something high performers avoid. Luckily, in this section, I am giving you tools to take control of your thoughts so you can command yourself to do anything, including getting up on your first alarm.

It takes emotions approximately five seconds to become convincing enough to influence action. With the Five Second Rule, you will beat your emotions to the decision by practicing acting before they take over. You can beat your emotions by creating a habit of making the logical decision before your feelings start taking control. Think of this exercise as working like a muscle: the more you practice it, the stronger it gets. At first you might not always beat your emotions; however, over time you will strengthen the ability to.

One key point is to know what outcome you want in advance. That way, it is not up for debate when it is time to act.

Let us apply the Five Second Rule to eating sweets. A lot of people wish they had more control over their sweet tooth. With the Five Second Rule, you can master the ability to control this temptation. All you have to do is two things: 1.) Decide on a sweet that is a non-negotiable. 2.) Replace the temptation with an immediate action. When you are confronted with the temptation, start counting down from five. Before the time is up, announce "No!" and physically walk away. The more exaggerated the announcement and maneuver the better. An exaggerated maneuver will convince your subconscious that you are serious. By following these two steps, you are making an immediate decision that there is no compromise. As a result, your mind will follow the actions of your body.

By practicing the Five Second Rule, you will develop the skill to always choose the beneficial option. You will teach yourself how to stop listening to your emotions and start listening to your mind. It is important for me to reiterate that you need to decide on the beneficial outcome in advance. An impulsive decision is not the right answer. I am not saying when you are debating large purchase and you are hesitating you should shut your feelings up and just buy it. I am saying, use the Five Second Rule to shut out emotions that are preventing you from growth. Over time, you will notice that you have a habit of always making the right decision over the emotional one.

In the book *Outliers*, Malcolm Gladwell states it takes approximately 10,000 hours to master a subject, and 66 days to establish a habit. Through awareness and practice, we can become masters of ourselves and develop the habits necessary for sustained growth.

Fortunately, humans have the ability to analyze our thoughts, and by using awareness, we can deliberately practice growth in all the three areas we just discussed. We can purposefully change our social environment, practice improving our genetic personality traits, and learn to control our emotional responses — ultimately becoming experts at managing ourselves.

Important to note is that results from making beneficial decisions are not usually immediate. You should feel rewarded for making choices that serve you, but you will not necessarily see the results until some time has passed.

Controlling our emotions takes time and practice. So does changing our social environment and modifying our personality traits. However, if you commit yourself to modifying these three categories, through compounding great decisions, you will achieve great results. Think of the small decisions like planting seeds in a garden. Every time you make a beneficial decision, you plant a seed. That seed needs time to grow. But if you continue to plant them, time will go by, and you will eventually have a beautiful garden.

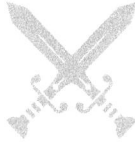

VISUALIZATION

*"Perfection is not attainable, but if we
chase it, we can achieve excellence."*
~ Vince Lombardi.

It is well known that professional athletes use visualization as a method to hone their skills and achieve excellence. In this first section of this book, we are focused on training the mind and changing how we think. Visualization is part of that training. You can use it to change what you think you are capable of and to keep you focused on what you want to achieve. I use visualization for many things, to include how I will act in military situational training exercises and combat. I have found that if I can visually rehearse conquering the upcoming mission, I am more likely to achieve success.

On the night before an operation, I will lie in bed and visually rehearse the plan. I will play out the sequence of events in great detail. I will think through all of the reports I need to give, the movement of the men working with me, and the actions I will take if/when we get in a gun fight. My goal is to practice what I want to accomplish in my mind before it happens. That way, I am becoming more effective on the battlefield before I get there. I visualize just like any professional athlete. It is a lot like rehearsing a football play or wresting match: I think through all of my actions and always finish the imagined scenario with what success looks like. I notice when I do not visualize, I am far more likely to fail.

The practice of visualizing will help you gravitate toward your goals. By keeping what you want in the forefront of your mind, you will develop laser-sharp focus of what you want to achieve. You will be less likely to get distracted and more likely to stay on course. I like to think of it like doing land navigation in the wilderness. Visualization is your azimuth (your true north) and the points you are after are your goals. When you are searching for a point, you need to pull out your compass to make sure you are on the correct course. Visualization will guide you and keep you focused on the direction in which you want to travel. If you do not pull out your compass, you will not have a clear image of where you are going. Without an azimuth, you will likely end up lost.

What I love about visualization is that you can use it for anything. Visualization helps build confidence, and confidence is paramount for success. It does not matter how you apply visualization. All that matters is that you build a habit of it. Whether you are trying to get in the best shape of your life or build wealth, visualization is another tool to keep you moving in the right direction.

It is typical for people to use visualization for sport but not life. Personally, I think most people do not know any better, or they are satisfied being a "goldfish." Luckily for you, you have become aware there is more to life than the bowl you live in, and you are taking action to improve yourself. At the end of this chapter, you will have another tool (visualization) to improve the way you think.

I have included visualization as part of the 12-week workout program later in this book. My recommendation is to start visualizing your fitness goals immediately. Picture yourself completing the program, developing your body, and training your mind. Visualize dominating each workout. Then, as you become more proficient, use visualization for other goals in life that you are after.

It is through focused routine visualization that I have been able to keep sight of my goals and achieve them. I have used it to accomplish my fastest ruck time of 1 hour and 57 minutes. To stay calm while being shot at, and to pass the U.S. Army Ranger School in one attempt. I am emphasizing the importance of visualization because it has done so much for me in my life, and I am hoping you adopt it as a method of achieving unprecedented heights.

I want to point out that it is important to not get stuck visualizing your worries and concerns. You should always visualize a positive outcome. Getting stuck thinking about failing is a recipe for failure. Your subconscious does not know the difference between a memory and an imagined scenario. To your subconscious, they both feel real. If you visualize failure too often, you will gravitate to it. You will be so focused on failure you will have no idea how to achieve success, so ensure you are visualizing positive images nested within accomplishing your goals. I am going to give you a breakdown of how I visualize so that you can develop your own method.

I typically visualize three times a day. Once in the morning, once after my workout, and once at night. I like to tie visualization to some sort of activity. Tying visualization to a physical action helps me keep it habitual and sustainable. I measure the success of the session by how I feel afterward. I know I have been successful when I open my eyes and can feel peace of mind and clarity. Those feelings give me the reward I need to keep practicing. I will generally visualize for 10 minutes each time. Ten minutes is a lot of time to imagine accomplishing your goals. It is sustainable and not too long to disrupt your day.

There is a saying: "If you do not have ten minutes, you do not have an hour." Meaning, everyone can find 10 minutes in their day, or they are just really bad at managing time.

If you want to start visualizing immediately (before you finish this book), start by setting a time today that you are going to do it. I recommend trying it before you go to bed. As you lie down and close your eyes, try this exercise.

Visualization Exercise

Before you go to sleep, end your night by thinking of your ideal future. You can imagine yourself in any future point in time — whether one year or 30-plus years. For simplicity in this exercise, imagine your future self in 10 years. Imagine the PERFECT DAY. Picture the entire day in extreme detail as if you have achieved your goals. Next, think of the actions you need to take tomorrow to build toward that dream.

Continue that process until you can play the images like a movie. Focus on the benchmarks that are important to you and visualize achieving all of them. Replay your movie from start to finish. Once you have created an entire decade of ideal images, repeat the process and expand the timeline. Visualize yourself toward the end of your life, happy and content with how you lived it. Imagine the feeling your achievements will bring, and bask in the feeling of winning.

Visualization takes practice. Some people will be able to do this exercise easier than others. If you struggle putting together the images in your mind, just be patient and keep practicing. At first you might get easily distracted or even fall asleep before you successfully imagine your full movie. However, through practice you will be able to visualize your future goals within seconds of starting.

Another way to help develop your visualization skills is to write out the "movie" in advance. It may seem time-consuming but writing out a script for accomplishing your goals is an investment. Writing out my goals is a routine that I exercise often. I like to do it three to four times a year so that I have a guide for my daily visualization. I write out what a perfect day entails to help with visualization. I write it in extreme detail, so that when I visualize, I have a detailed image embedded into my memory, and I can go back and reread any areas that are unclear. If you spend 30 minutes writing out your goals in detail, you can spend the next year or more rehearsing it in your mind before bed. An example of me reaching my goals in writing starts like this:

"I wake up, no alarm needed, I'm eager for the day. I am a bit groggy. My feet move off the bed and to the carpet. A soft rug is under my feet. I feel tired, but eager for the day ahead. I drop to my knees and begin my prayer. After, I kiss my wife and move to my beautiful kitchen to turn on the coffee. I can smell the grounds. My home is on the beach, and I can hear the waves. After cleansing my body with a glass of water, I go to my desk and read the news. It is 3:20am and I am ahead of the rest of the world. I have a lot ahead of me. A workout and growing my business are on my priority list. I walk down the stairs of my beautiful home and into my gym. I turn the gym lights on and appreciate how far I have come...."

I continue writing that "movie" for the entire day. I highlight the parts that bring me the most pleasure. When I lay down at night, I visually rehearse the details and accomplishments I wrote. I picture loved ones' faces around me. I picture life as I reach my highest potential. As you continue to practice, your visualizations will become closer and closer to reality. You will naturally drift toward the life you are mentally rehearsing. It has happened to me numerous times. Moments that I have previously visualized seem to coincidentally appear.

Through repeated visualization, you will begin to get confident in what you can accomplish. The compounding effects will help you stay ambitious and focused. Continue to practice visualization daily with the intention of getting 1% better. It will not be long before you reach unprecedented heights.

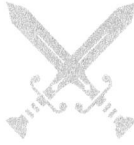

LAW OF ATTRACTION MANIFESTING COMBAT

"Where focus goes energy flows."
~ Tony Robbins.

If you are anything like I used to be, you might roll your eyes at the title of this chapter; however, I have become a big believer in the Law of Attraction. For those unfamiliar, the Law of Attraction is a theory that states we will receive things equitable to how we think and feel. It is founded on the premise that by focusing on an outcome, you will set in motion events that will materialize that desire. For example, if you constantly think and feel that you are out of shape, you will continue to act in that manner. As a result, you will "manifest" an out-of-shape body. In contrast, if you start to think and feel like you are an athlete, you will become one.

I have included a section on the Law of Attraction because it is a tool I used to manifest some of my deepest desires. I have used it in the past to manifest combat and achieve my goals. By reading this section on "The Law of Attraction" you will increase your ability to accomplish your goals. It is one more tool to help shape the way you think. In the previous chapter, I taught you how to use visualization to gravitate you toward your goals. In this section, you will learn how the Law of Attraction will gravitate your goals to you.

I heard about the Law of Attraction in 2006 when a known book titled *The Secret, by Rhonda Byrne,* was released. People everywhere criticized it, and to be fair, I did too. I thought the idea of miraculously manifesting something I wanted was ridiculous. I even cracked a joke about manifesting ice cream. I pretended I was going to use "The Secret" to make ice cream appear in front of me. When it did not work, I confidently announced how I had disproved the theory.

Years later, I began to have a different opinion. I remember the day my opinions of the Law of Attraction changed. I was deployed at the time and had just come back from a mission. My platoon had spent the night conducting a capture/kill mission and had just got back to our living quarters. I lay down in bed after all the post-mission requirements were complete and thought back through everything that had happened. We had gotten into an intense firefight, and had accomplished the mission. As I lay in bed, it came to my realization everything that I just experienced, I had first visualized years before. Some of those experiences included the terrain we traveled in, the faces of those fighting next to me, and the movement of individuals on the battlefield. The feeling that I had manifested that mission was unreal. Before that moment, I had no idea I was practicing the Law of Attraction regularly. So how did I do it? Let me tell you how it started in the example below.

In 2009, I made the decision to switch from an enlisted soldier to officer in the Army. I decided I was going to go back to college after dropping out four years prior. I was utterly disappointed with my life and wanted to go back to school to finish what I had started. I took my first leap of faith and applied for the Army's Green to Gold Scholarship Program.

I did not think I was going to get in, but I knew I was at least going to try. To my utter surprise, my application was approved. At this point, I was not set on joining the Infantry, I was focused on getting my college education. I thought that I would get my degree and come back into the Army as an engineer. However, my interest changed.

Getting accepted into the Army's Green to Gold Program increased my confidence and I began thinking I was capable of achieving more. I started developing a "who cares? I am going for it anyway" attitude. As soon as I got to college, I found myself gravitating toward the mental and physical toughness challenges to make it into the Army's elite units. In my mind, I had nothing to lose. I had already lived a life I was not pleased with, so I decided to allow myself to pursue a path that inspired me.

It was during my third term in college when I felt like a career in combat arms was my calling. I made the decision to compete for a competitive slot to commission as an Infantry Officer. Simultaneously, I began to get excited about the unknown and the adventure on which this new path would take me. I began to develop an insatiable desire to prove myself in combat as an infantryman. After three years of working on my goal, I graduated college and made it into the infantry.

To my disappointment, the fighting overseas at this time was fading. Increasingly, my peers were getting less time on combat assignments. It was beginning to look like I would never get a chance to prove myself as an Infantryman like I had set out to. Regardless, every night I lay down, I visualized how I would act in a firefight. I visualized how I would handle my emotions, and how I would control them on the battlefield. I stubbornly believed that regardless of the experiences of others, I would eventually be tested. I continued to visualize my ultimate desires in detail.

It was at this moment that the Law of Attraction began to take action. As my career progressed, I naturally gravitated toward my goal. I made incremental gains toward my desires to fight in combat. The first benchmark was when I graduated Infantry Basic Officer Leader Course. The next was making it into the 75th Ranger Regiment. I spent years practicing the Law of Attraction through visualization.

To my surprise, years later, I found myself living the exact moments I had visualized. Not just the general concept, but *exact* situations and sequences of events. The unique part is that I thought of these events years before I was in a combat arms occupation. At the time, they were manifestations of my desire to win, prove myself, and make a difference. Little did I know, one day the scenarios I had pictured would unfold in front of me. I truly believe it was the Law of Attraction that pulled me toward living those exact moments. Living that exact situation was an impossible thing to plan beforehand.

It was outside of my control. However, despite the odds, I was blessed with living out my deepest desires.

It never occurred to me that by visualizing I was bringing my deepest desires to reality. The night that I lay in bed reflecting on the scenario I had imagined years before, it occurred to me that I had been using the Law of Attraction since I was a child. My earliest occurrence began in the third grade. The older students were putting the biographies of the younger students into the yearbook. I told them that I wanted to be in the U.S. Army when I grew up. As I got older, the idea of joining the military never crossed my mind again. In fact, I told the recruiter when I was in high school that I would never join. I dodged him for months. I was disgusted at his salesman pitches and cheesy pep talks. I refused to join the Army and decided I would give college a chance. I attended two semesters at a community college and quickly dropped out. I had no clear path in life and I did not enjoy the day-to-day lifestyle.

I was lost and had no direction as to where I wanted to go with my life. So guess what option I chose? I gave in and signed a contract to enlist into the Army. Then a few years later, I was visiting my parents when my brother walked up to me with my elementary school yearbook. He opened it up and showed me my interview from the third grade. I was shocked. In the yearbook I said that when I grew up, I wanted to join the Army.

At nineteen years old, I ended up in the exact place I had wanted to when I was eight. I had attracted the future I once imagined and desired. It might have been a coincidence, but it also could have been the Law of Attraction.

There are a few theories on how the Law of Attraction works. My belief is that the Law of Attraction is emotion-based — that the feelings you carry cause subtle actions that draw in the specific outcome on which you are focused.

The Law of Attraction will gravitate you closer to your passions and your worries. Whenever you are focused on an outcome, you send subconscious messages to your soul. Those subconscious messages program you to work every day toward the outcome you are imagining. Then, when your brain is on autopilot, you make mindless decisions that stack up until those desires are brought to fruition.

In order to channel the Law of Attraction, focus on the pleasurable feelings of getting what you want. If you want to be in better shape, carry the feeling of being in shape. Use visualization exercises like in the previous chapter to generate those feelings. You will notice that through repetition and practice, you will begin to attract a fit lifestyle. The Law of Attraction is generally pretty simple. Thoughts lead to emotions and emotions lead to actions. Therefore, carry the emotions that will draw you toward the desired outcome.

If you want to learn more, read *The Law of Attraction*, by Michael Losier. His book is by far the best resource I have found to learn how to use the Law of Attraction correctly. Additionally, Sarah Centrella's book *Hustle, Believe, Receive* is a great resource. She interviews 51 people in different stages of their life and reveals how each of them achieved their goals through the Law of Attraction. I recommend both books to supplement this program. Learning how to manifest your desires in a physical capacity will put you on a trajectory you never thought possible.

The Law of Attraction is part of this program because the power of it starts with your thoughts. What we think about attracts what we get. The Law of Attraction is another tool to help you on your journey toward a higher level of performance. Like all of the tools I am providing you, apply them to fitness first. When you get to the workout program, visualize your body developing over the course of the next 12 weeks. Focus on the results you want, not the results you do not. Record your progress and watch the Law of Attraction transform your thoughts into reality.

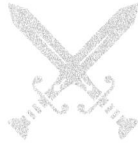

ROUTINES

"Plan your life with a vision and your day by the clock."
~ Zig Ziglar

N ow that we have discussed ways to shift your thinking and work toward your goals, it is time to build a routine to ensure sustained growth. The workout program at the end of this book includes a physical routine — a routine structured for building your body. In the next couple of chapters, I am going to discuss daily routines to help you train outside of exercising.

Routines and rituals give us the power to control our day and our future. Routines can help produce massive amounts of productivity or keep us stagnant. They can be the difference between feeling accomplished and looking back at the last 10 years and wondering why we have not moved forward. They enable us to get the most out of our day. With a simple routine, we can be proactive with our time, gaining traction that would be otherwise lost to reactivity and unpreparedness.

In any occupation, work can be time-consuming. Serving in the military is no exception. When I was in the 75th Ranger Regiment, it was common to work 20- to 22-hour days for multiple days at a time. I would have limited time to pursue my personal goals because of the demands of my job. I decided to design a routine that allowed me to accomplish more with my limited time. I analyzed the things that were important to me and came up with a plan to have more time for them. Instead of complaining about the lack of time, I decided to listen to the words of Zig Ziglar, "You can't make more time but you can make better use of it."

I structure each day around the idea of "chunking." Chunking is a term used to describe how your brain groups information so that you remember it. During high-stress situations, the brain is only able to recall an average of three things. It uses chunking to do so effectively.

Chunking is the reason phone numbers are broken into three parts. Why "stop, drop, and roll" consists of three key actions. And why 9-1-1 is three numbers long. Chunking is a way to take complex information and group it into ways that the brain will remember. It works for remembering things and it is also a great starting point for structuring a day.

Using the chunking concept, I divide my day into three parts: personal, professional, and personal. A typical day for me starts with personal time and ends with personal time. Personal time includes any activity outside of the job I currently work. Some examples include meditation, reading, and other goals like working on this book. Professional time includes anything related to my career. For most, it is their 9-to-5.

The amount of time spent in each of these designations is relative to the amount of time available. If "professional" time takes up 16 hours out of my day, then I am left with eight hours of "personal" time. I typically break up the available hours of personal time to rest and make progress outside of my 9-to-5. If I have eight hours of personal time available, I will sleep for six, work on this book for one, and have one hour of family time. Chunking creates more time for things that are important to me. Notably, the chunking structure is scalable. If I finish with my professional work early (say within four hours) then I have 20 hours for personal time, and it is up to me how to use them.

When building your daily routine, try applying the "chunking" concept to your day. After you break up your day into personal and professional time (or whatever reflects your current situation), list out what you want to accomplish in each part then implement a plan to achieve it. Block off the morning and evening for your personal goals and allow the middle of your day to be consumed with work. If you are not sure where to start, that is OK. In the next chapter, I will show you an example of my morning and evening routines so you have a template to mirror if you choose.

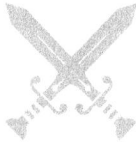

MORNING ROUTINES

"There is no change without a change in routine."
~ Tai Lopez

Have you ever had a day where everything went your way? Where you stacked up win after win as if you were unstoppable? That momentum is exactly what a morning routine can do. A structured morning routine provides the opportunity to start your day working on your goals and doing what is most important. As you accomplish your goals, you will start to build confidence you can do more. Over time, that combination of confidence and achievement will compound into massive momentum. Simply put, morning routines are a formula for success.

One of the things I love about mornings are they are the one time of the day that is under our control. We can always wake up earlier – before distractions and obligations.

However, I did not always think like that. Like a lot of people, I used to wake up and react to life instead of being proactive toward it. Over time, I learned that having a process that generates momentum early in the day allowed to me to make more progress. I learned this lesson when I was training for the 75th Ranger Regiment. I structured my day using the chunking concept (previously discussed) and blocked off personal time before work. Trying to work on my goals while I was at work was completely unfeasible. I used the time to train physically and mentally for the upcoming selection. I read, visualized, and exercised prior to stepping into my first meeting of the day. I would wake up at 0400 and complete as many personal tasks as possible until 0600. Repeating that behavior every day for months set me up for success at the selection. I was accepted into the 75th Ranger Regiment because I prepared well.

Morning routines come with obstacles. Getting up before you absolutely have to is one of them. Right now, the idea of getting up earlier probably sounds painful. Trust me, I can relate. My first meeting of the day usually starts at 0600, and I generally need to be at work at 0530. Creating personal time while it is still dark out does not sound appealing. But if you create a simple morning routine that serves you, you will be far more likely to accomplish your goals.

If waking up is difficult for you, then front-load your morning with an activity that you enjoy. Find an incentive that gives you energy and pleases you. Coffee and reading are my incentives. When I am tired, convincing myself to get up for a cup of coffee and a chapter of my book is a lot easier than telling myself to get up for a 20-mile run.

Morning routines should be tailored toward YOUR goals. You cannot become an accountant by studying biology. You cannot reach the pinnacle of your ideas of success using someone else's routines. To help build sustainable habits, nest personal goals into the habits you are going to repeat every morning. Gain control of the morning and start WINNING early. I tackle my morning routine by using a simple framework: Prep the Body, Prep the Mind, Tend to the Soul.

Prep the Body

As soon as my alarm goes off, I give myself five seconds to drop off the bed and to my knees. When my knees hit the floor, I have control of my body. From my knees, I pray and give gratitude. Expressing gratitude for the simple things in my life is a way to immediately begin the day with positivity and appreciation. Once I finish praying, I make the bed. It is not perfect, but I toss my side of the covers over and make sure it looks neat. I abide by the message of Navy Seal Admiral William H. McRaven, who said, "Making your bed is a way to accomplish the first task of the day, and one task turns into accomplishing two tasks...." He continued to say, "...and if you have a miserable day, at least you come back to a bed you made, it'll give you encouragement tomorrow will be better." After the bed is made and my first tasks are complete, I brush my teeth. While brushing, I recite in my mind the goals I have written on my bathroom mirror. I continue to express gratitude and give thanks for life. Approximately 151,000 people die each day, so waking up is a miracle and success in itself. For that I am thankful. After brushing my teeth, I splash cold water on my face to change my state. Cold water will charge your central nervous system and change your body's chemistry to an alert state.

Next, I move to my kitchen for a glass of water to give myself an "inner bath." I learned this from *The Model Health Show* host Shawn Stevenson. While I'm drinking a glass of water, I continue to think of all the things I am grateful for and what I am excited about. When the glass is empty, I drop to the floor and do five pushups. Why five pushups? Five is an easy number; on my worst day, I can knock out five pushups with very little effort. It is a simple way to add another win to the day using healthy habits. When I knock out five pushups in the morning as an old man, I will feel young and healthy. After my five pushups, I turn on the coffee machine and move to my desk to begin the second stage of my morning.

Prep the Mind

I prep my mind by reading. I pick up a book, and use the messages to prompt introspection. Typically I like to read some sort of history or philosophy in the morning. Recently, I completed *The Daily Stoic*, which includes 366 meditations on stoicism. The short chapters are a page in length and give valuable insight. I always consider the ways the lessons apply to me, and I determine what I can take away from the passages. I think it is important to collect the various lessons that surround us. They are all around us, and by finding them early in my day I have something to focus on to better my mindset and make me a better person. After I finish my reading, I am ready for my first cup of coffee.

Alongside my morning coffee, I pull out my affirmations and recite out loud all the beliefs I am trying to instill into my subconscious. The affirmations are written in such a way that I believe them and feel them in my soul. Once I finish my affirmations, I transition to my daily journal entry. Journaling has a few specific purposes in my life. The main purpose is to annotate growth and record the lessons I have acquired from the previous day. This practice helps keep me focused on my end state and making steady progress. Also, if I have any nagging thoughts, I can use this journaling to analyze and dispose of destructive thought patterns and move forward with my intentions for the day. The key to journaling is to do it before any outside influence.

I have not yet touched my phone at this point in my routine. It is important for me to get to this point of my morning without checking texts, emails, or social media, so that I can journal without influence. Distractions only cloud my thoughts and influence what I write. Therefore, I try to keep journaling as pure as possible by doing so with a clear mind.

I spend about 10 to 15 minutes journaling. On the mornings I am thoughtless, I sustain the habit and simply write down that there was not anything on my mind. I do everything in my power to at least record one word or sentence so that I never lose the routine.

After journaling, I transition to the final stage of my morning: "Tend to the soul."

Tend to the Soul

I tend to the soul every morning by meditating and exercising. After I journal, I sit down on the floor and cross my legs. I reserve 10 minutes to meditate each morning. I prefer to sit on the ground because I believe there is a correlation between fitness and our relationship to the ground. Most people avoid the ground. They prop themselves up to put on their shoes, they sit in chairs, and never really interact with it. In fact, most people avoid it. Meditating on the floor gives me an opportunity to assess my physical mobility. If I can get onto and off the floor easily, then I know have been stretching enough.

Once I get set on the floor, I begin meditating. I use two techniques. In the first, I try to focus on having empty thoughts. In the second technique, I allow my mind to wander and explore whatever path it leads me on. I start both by focusing on my breath and then shifting my focus to one of the two techniques. I have found meditation brings calmness and clarity into my life. Additionally, it has numerous health benefits. It decreases stress levels and increases the density of grey matter in your brain. Increased grey matter has a positive effect on memory and learning. Additionally, a regular meditation practice allows an opportunity to reset my mind before I leave the house.

I began using apps and guided meditations when I first started. But I created my own system as I learned what was effective for me. If you want to add meditating to your morning routine, I highly suggest the phone application called Headspace. Headspace offers a free trial period so you can determine if it is for you. They charge around $10 a month to keep your subscription. They offer various categories like Focus, Health, Motivation, and Sport for your choosing. I personally used their app for a year before I branched off and started my own method.

After I have meditated, I head out the door for my morning workout. Exercising in the morning puts me into a confident state and removes any stress that I may have. Additionally, I like to use working out as a method of personal development. I will share how I do this in the workout section. To put it simply, I will capture lessons from podcasts and books periodically throughout my week and use exercising as a method to act on those lessons. For instance, I was listening to Andy Frisella's podcast the other day on "Arete" – meaning excellence in all you do. The message was that we should treat everything with "Arete." I adapted the lesson and applied it to my workout. I was doing intervals at the time, and every time I increased my effort, I chanted the mantra "Arete!" It became a method of building the idea of excellence into my subconscious. I like to have one lesson per workout, and I focus on it with the intention of training my body and mind at the same time.

The current mantra of my workouts is "Go just a little bit further." Dominick Cruz stated that his talent lies in his ability to go past the level where most people quit. I took this message to heart and applied it to my workouts. This means every measure of effort this week is about going past where I would normally quit and doing "just a little bit more." As the workout progresses, endorphins are released and the mindset becomes more believable. I start to feel confident that "I always go just a little bit further." The message has become believable, and it travels with me throughout my day. I try to keep the same theme for a few consecutive days to really establish it into my beliefs.

I think I have been successful throughout my military career because of the way I train the body and mind simultaneously. I believe training them together gives me an edge over others who do not. When I was training for selection for the 75th Ranger Regiment, I would repeatedly use the lesson: "I am good enough." That mantra gave me the confidence I needed to break past my fear of failure.

I have included the lessons I've found the most effective in the workout program of this book. These are the lessons that I continue to fall back on to sustain growth and progress. Feel free to add, subtract, and/or change them to suit you. Use them as a guide in your morning routine to train yourself both mentally and physically.

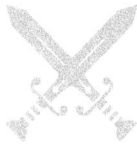

EVENING ROUTINES

"Set the set piece before you move the move piece."
~ Military Philosophy

This is a quote I picked up in the military while learning to synchronize multiple assets during combat. It emphasizes not moving your "pieces" before the appropriate time, also known as "setting the conditions." It is the final check on all men, weapons, and equipment to make sure that all of your combat power is prepared and ready to be used on the objective.

Setting the conditions gives you an unfair advantage for the purpose of WINNING. It encompasses both diligence and preparation to ensure tasks are completed correctly. Those are precisely the tools we will use to attack our evening routine.

The framework for an evening routine is:

1.   Prepare Yourself

2. Reward Yourself

3. Transition Yourself

What I love most about the framework for the evening routine is that it directly correlates to methods used in the U.S. Army's Ranger School. For those unfamiliar, Ranger School is a 62-day course that evaluates individual infantry tactics and leadership. Service members who go through are sleep-deprived and tested continuously through three phases.

During the course, each Ranger candidate rotates into and out of leadership positions and gets evaluated on their performance. Rangers march until late hours of the night and complete missions. When the last mission of the day is complete, it is time for them to prepare for the next day. They prepare their weapons and equipment, then reward themselves with a Meal, Ready-to-Eat (MRE), and finally transition to a rest cycle. Patrols will often go past 0200 in the morning with Rangers waking up at 0400. It is imperative that all members set the conditions before they bed down. They must prepare for the next day and have everything staged to maximize performance and to prepare for any contingencies that may arise.

Prepare Yourself

Preparation is the first step for the evening routine. It can take the body two to three hours to become efficient in thinking and performing after a night of sleep. I build my evening routing to streamline the first few hours of the day. I do this to take the load off the cognitive mind and make the morning efficient. Every night before you start winding down, ask yourself, "What do I need to do to 'set the conditions' for tomorrow?" It could be writing the key tasks you have for the next day, laying out your gym clothes, or completing your meal prep. Consider each night what pieces need to be put in the correct position in order to overwhelm and destroy tomorrow.

Reward Yourself

Once you have completed all of your key tasks and prepared for the next day, you should feel complete. Feeling complete is one of my favorite tools to assess the day. If I am honest with myself, I know when I have given the day my all. The feeling of it being complete is unique.

When I accomplish that feeling, it is time for a reward. Positive reinforcement is an effective way to make a habit sustainable. The reward is relative to the individual. For some, it could be an activity. For others, a conversation, or perhaps quiet time. For me, a nightly reward usually consists of connecting with a person close to me.

Rewards at the end of the day do two things: they reinforce the positive act of being productive, and they give you something to look forward to. They are also scalable. The more my productivity, the bigger my reward. I use Friday as my reward night. If I win the week, I plan an activity for Friday evening. Now, I know what a lot of you are thinking... "What about drinking?" Well, I'll tell you that drinking depends on the individual and that's your decision to make. Remember our focus is "setting the conditions" for the next day in order to optimize performance. I have experimented with drinking and for me, personally, it does not work; it takes away from my confidence and sets the next day up for failure. However, do as you wish. My recommendation is to try several things to discover what works and does not work.

Transition Yourself

Transitioning into a resting state should be a system developed to expedite the process of falling asleep while also ensuring deep rest. I have pulled some of my night routine from peak performance expert, thought leader, and decamillionaire, Ed Mylett. He is a big believer in using a "warm" theme to transition at night. Adding warm elements to your environment triggers the body to relax. Warm baths work great, as does warm tea. Pick a relaxing activity like reading a fiction book or journaling for pleasure to get control of your mind and shut off the problem-solving processes. Once you have decompressed, it is time to enter "disciplined sleep." We will talk about sleep in the next section but is important to note the importance of enforcing a strict sleeping routine.

Sticking to a specified bedtime will keep you operating at a high level. The amount of sleep each individual needs is controversial; however, if you study exceptional businessmen, entrepreneurs, and anyone elite in their field, you will notice very few of them get more than six hours of sleep a night. In contrast, professional athletes often advocate for eight or more hours of sleep. Tom Brady, for example, is a firm believer in nine hours of sleep. He calls it "regeneration time."

I am going to offer six hours of sleep *as a guide.* If you need more than that, go ahead, just know that there are individuals out there who have trained themselves to sleep less. In the end, remember, all of this is about performance. Calculate your sleep based on how you operate the best. Condensing sleep takes practice just like growing a muscle. If you start cutting off too much at once, your body is going to have a tough time keeping up. Instead, identify the target number of hours you want to achieve (your goal) and shave off a little bit each night until you accomplish it.

While you are training yourself to sleep less, continue to transition yourself for the next day. Include 10-15 minutes for visualizations while in bed. Start by visualizing all the things you are grateful for — start small and express gratitude for the things that are unique to you. One of the unique, small things for which I am personally grateful is my bed. I have slept in a lot of strange places while being in the military. Expressing gratitude for the simple comforts I have nightly reinforces a positive mindset that serves me.

After you have thought through what you are grateful for, play the mental movie you created in the visualization chapter. Play out your future expectations and goals in your mind's eye. Visualize in detail the next day, week, month, and year. Visualize accomplishment while you transition to a full night's rest.

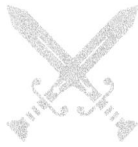

SLEEP MASTERING PERFORMANCE

"An idle mind is the devil's playground…
unless you master the playground."
~ Jeramiah Solven

E fficient sleep is a key tool for optimizing performance. Proper sleep gives you more energy to dominate the next day, and that is exactly what this book is about. Sleep, or the lack thereof, is a huge issue in the United States. Sleep deprivation is quickly becoming an epidemic. Why is it common to ask somebody how they are doing, and have them respond with "Oh, I'm tired"?

The reasons are: 1.) Like attracts like, and feeling tired is more often a mindset than a reality. 2.) Most people do not know HOW to sleep. A lot of people are taught to fall asleep through distraction, be it a television, drinking, cell phones, or medication. The solution isn't in any of these "Band-Aids"; the solution is in practicing behaviors that encourage deep and restful sleep. The ability to fall asleep is just like a muscle. It takes repetition to grow the muscle and discipline to stay consistent. What makes sleeping without distractions hard is that we are forced to deal with the pain that exists in all of our minds. Pain can stem from a variety of sources, like past experiences or future anxiety. Even the preconceived notion that we might have a difficult time falling asleep can be enough to keep us up.

I personally used to dislike going to bed. Sleeping was difficult for me because my brain would race before bed. When I lay down, my mind would begin to rapid-fire about the future, the past, what I needed to do, and what I might have forgotten. Because of the problems I had with sleep, I have spent countless hours researching the topic and trying different methods to achieve a good night's rest. I have experimented with several over-the-counter aids, alcohol, and teas, none of which have enabled me to operate at 100% the next day. After practice and mental reframing, I have been able to conquer sleep, and now I look forward to it. The methods I used that solved my sleeping problems and allowed me to wake up fully rested and energized for the day were: 1.) Create a sleep sanctuary. 2.) Create an enjoyable experience. 3.) Understand your chronotype.

1.) Create a sleep sanctuary

Your bedroom should be a place designed for comfort and relaxation — a sanctuary of sorts. I highly recommend buying curtains that allow you to make it as dark as a cave and block out sound. Additionally, limit your activities in your bedroom to sleeping. Too many people have televisions in their bedrooms, and electronics screaming for attention throughout the night. Get rid of as many distractions as you can. This includes light. Light omits currents that limit the amount of the hormone melatonin your body releases.

Melatonin is a naturally occurring hormone in your body that convinces you to be tired. Preventing light exposure encourages melatonin release. Adjust the settings on your cell phone to block out early in the night and to get tired sooner. Most phones have a night setting that cuts out the blue light omitting from the screen and tricks your body's photoreceptors into releasing melatonin. Light and sound are your enemy in your sleep sanctuary, so you need to destroy them at all costs.

Lastly, your bed should be the most expensive piece of furniture in your home; it should feel like heaven. It is the final place you visit before you dominate the next day. I read that most people spend one third of their life in their beds, so give it the respect it deserves. Invest in a nice mattress and keep a nice comfortable blanket with you if you travel. I keep a deployment blanket with me when I go overseas. My current one has a tiger on it and is as soft as the clouds. I cannot help but laugh every time I think of a "tough infantryman" cuddled up in his nice deployment blanket. Now, if you are on a tight budget, start with quality sheets and covers and just slowly upgrade the quality of your bed over time.

2.) Create an enjoyable experience

Falling asleep should be something about which you are excited. Look at falling asleep as an opportunity to rehearse visualization and dream about your future goals. We have talked about the power of visualization in this book, and practicing it as a part of your evening routine will give you something to look forward to. Instead of stressing about what you cannot control at night, focus on what you can: your thoughts. If you are struggling to build a rewarding experience, revisit the chapter on evening routines. Specifically, review the "warm" concept mentioned. A warm bath or warm tea can help create a positive nightly experience. If those do not do the trick, maybe a non-fiction book will. The enjoyable experience you create should be planned and timed. Without structure, it is far more likely that you will fall into a routine of whatever everyone else in your house is doing, which can be sabotaging if their activities do not serve you.

3.) Understand your chronotype

Point number three of attaining efficient sleep is to have an understanding of your chronotype. I use the word 'chronotype' to convey the idea of knowing your propensity to sleep at a certain point in the day. You should have an understanding of the time of the day when you are most tired and energized. Take note of the times of the day you operate the best so that you can build a routine that is natural for you.

The Power of When, written by Dr. Michael Breus and Dr. Mehmet Oz is an amazing book that discusses how everyone's genes can dictate the time windows in which they perform best. He categorizes people into animal types (lions, bears, dolphins, and wolves), and goes into detail about how each animal operates efficiently at certain times throughout the day. For example, he says that society is generally tailored towards 'bears'. Bears make up the 50-55% of society who naturally wake up and go to bed when the sun rises and sets. They are most efficient around 10:00 to 11:00 am. What is important is to understand not everyone is an early riser genetically. Understanding which "animal" you are will give you an assessment of how you should design your day. It will help you determine if you should wake up early and go to bed early or if you should wake up later and stay up later.

Dr. Breus has a quiz online you can take to discover your animal doppelganger (thepowerofwhenquiz.com). Learn about what animal you are so that you can stop comparing yourself to the other animals in the kingdom and capitalize on who you are efficiently.

Getting a good night's rest also comes down to responding productively when your sleep is interrupted. If you have the right tools to deal with it, interrupted sleep does not have to be stressful. Some tools to use to fall back asleep are: reading, more visualization, or a paradoxical intention. A paradoxical intention is one of my favorites because of its effectiveness, and I find it fun to play tricks on the mind. A paradoxical intention means telling yourself you want a certain outcome so that you receive the opposite. It would be like telling yourself you can have all the cookies in the world so that you can stop thinking about not having them.

An example of a paradoxical intention is found in the book *A Man's Search For Meaning* by Victor Frankl. Victor Frankl was an author and psychologist who survived the Holocaust. He wrote about treating patients with insomnia. He states that the fear of insomnia will cause "anticipatory anxiety" and the person will hyper-intend to fall asleep, which means they will try too hard to fall asleep. One method used in treatment is to cause the patient to redirect the obsession and interrupt the worry of not sleeping with the idea they have the choice to get up.

I adopted the technique of creating a paradoxical intention with sleep. I will close my eyes and telling myself I can get up if I want to. I will also tell myself to open my eyes if I am "as wide awake" as I think I am. As soon as I hear that message, my mind becomes focused on how tired I actually am. The little voice in my head starts convincing me that I do not actually want to be awake. The next thing you know, I am less stressed out about the idea of not getting any sleep. I soon become more tired, and shortly after, I am sound asleep.

Lastly, when I notice I am not sleeping well, I take a close look at my patterns and behaviors. Not sleeping properly usually comes down to two things: I slept too much the night before, or I did not give the day my maximum effort. Analyzing my sleep gives me the ability to refine the process. Adjusting my sleep and how hard I applied myself in the day are two methods to ensure a good night sleep. For me, personally, If I get more than six hours of sleep a night I will have difficulty falling asleep. If six hours is not enough for you, think of the joke from Arnold Schwarzenegger, who said: "All you need is six hours of sleep. If you need more, just sleep a little faster."

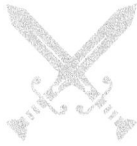

TIME MANAGEMENT

*"You cannot make more time but you
can make better use of it."*
~ Unknown

Everyone I know struggles with time, and it is up to us to master it. I have learned in the military that if we want to achieve massive results, we need to focus our effort on effectiveness over efficiency.

Tim Ferriss, author of *The 4-Hour Work Week*, best described the comparison of these two. He stated that efficiency is doing all the right things, while effectiveness is doing all the right things well. I love the concept of effectiveness because it is results-based. It is about getting the most out of your effort and time. People assume the most beneficial way of trying to get more than one thing done at a time is to multitask. Multitasking can be efficient, but it is never effective. Multitasking is a made-up concept adopted by humans during the invention of computers. Computers had the ability to switch between two tasks so quickly that it seemed as if they were accomplishing them simultaneously. Humans adopted the ability to multitask as a skill to be lauded. But in truth, multitasking is just doing two things poorly. Allow me to reshape the way you think about time so that you can become more effective with it.

The human brain only has the ability to focus on one thing at a time. The contrarians reading this right now are arguing: "Well, I can listen to music and write a paper at the same time; that is doing TWO things!" My response is that you are not effectively listening to the music and that is why you are able to focus on the paper. If the task was to listen to every word in a new song and write the paper, could you? The answer is no.

A more effective way of achieving a result is to do what is called "task stacking." Task stacking is using multiple independently operating resources to reach a desired outcome. Think of getting your hair cut and your boots shined. In task stacking, you would have one person cut your hair, and one person shine your shoes. The end result would be that your shoes are well shined, and your hair is well cut. Now in multitasking you would try to cut your hair and shine your shoes yourself. It would take twice as much time to complete as task stacking. And you would just end up with messed up boots and a poor haircut.

Task stacking is the method I use to consume information. It is the reason I am able to read and/or listen to a book a week. It is also the reason I can listen to five hours of podcasts a week. A couple ways to implement stack task involve transportation and exercise. Whenever you have the opportunity to ride in the passenger seat, take advantage of it. Open your book or turn on your audio. You will be moving toward your destination and making progress reading. Driving yourself and listening to audiobooks is efficient, but listening while riding as a passenger is *effective*. In the passenger seat, you can actively listen and take notes. Retention is far higher when you are able to focus on just the one task.

Another example of task stacking is in exercise. As I transition to my workout for the day, my warmup and stretching routine is stacked with an audiobook or podcast. I give myself enough time to write down notes. I will start by walking on the treadmill and taking notes. The walk is an independent task since it requires no thought. My warmups and cooldowns usually take 15-30 minutes a day. These habits allow me to consume over five hours of information weekly. The walking and stretching example is close to multitasking; however, I still consider it task stacking because of how unconscious the skill of walking is.

Another way to think of effectiveness is to understand how it works in combat. Imagine conducting a raid on a compound and you have 50 motivated, intelligent soldiers and nothing else. There is a single guy inside of a house and you want to clear it and capture him alive (the result). If you were limited to having ground soldiers only, efficiency would allow you to place your soldiers around the compound and then to clear it from one end to the next. If each solider is proficient in their job, they can act smoothly and quickly. However, if the bad guy runs, even in the most efficient scenario, it may take several minutes (if not hours) for the ground force soldiers to chase him down.

Now view the scenario through the lens of effectiveness. Equip the ground force of 50 motivated soldiers with a helicopter and interdiction team (independent resources). The helicopter's task is to watch the compound and transport the team on board to capture any bad guy who flees. When the target flees in this scenario, the ground force continues to clear the house and the helicopter touches down near-simultaneously to intercept the runner. The result is the target is captured within moments. Effectiveness over efficiency always wins.

Another method I use to get the most out of my time is by changing my mindset to get two days out of one. This might sound a bit odd to some, but I convince myself there are two days in a 24-hour period. I divide my day into two eight-hour periods. This concept ends up giving me (mentally) 14 days in a week when everyone else is only operating with seven. The trick is to realize there is more to the day then the 9-5 that most people live by. The first part of my day goes from 0400 until 1200. The second part goes from 1230 to 2030. The remaining two hours I will spend awake are for family time and resetting for the next day.

In the middle of the day, I like to give myself a 30-minute "transition period." I like to implement a short break in the middle of the day to recharge my mind and body. The goal is to take a break so that I can tackle the rest of my day with as much energy as the first. I deliberately DO NOT call it a "rest period." The idea of resting puts the brain in a more relaxed state, which can easily become a habit of laziness. Instead, I think of it like a break between missions. I know that after the transition point, I am going back to the objective.

This transition period includes 30 minutes of planned mindless activity. Meditation or listening to music are great examples. The transition period should include a short routine that gets you operating back at one hundred percent. "What about naps?" you ask. I have experimented with naps, but unless I am running on fewer than six hours of sleep, I prefer not to. I have found it takes me too long to bring myself back to optimal operating speed after a nap. which takes a toll on my effectiveness for the remainder of the day. Two of my favorite things to do during my transition period are to catch up on texts and talk briefly to loved ones. At the end of the transition period, I like to reward myself with a coffee or refreshing drink to charge me into the next leg of the day.

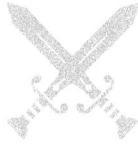

DISCIPLINE

"Discipline equals freedom."
~ Jocko Willink

etired Navy Seal Jocko Willink believes that discipline is the solution for freedom. And that through applied discipline, you can achieve anything. I absolutely agree with his belief. That is why I think it is important to include how to build discipline in this book. We can develop it like any muscle in our bodies — practicing a little bit at a time until we have unbelievable strength. There are three techniques that I use to practice and build discipline: 1.) Preserve the fuel 2.) Make it a critical task. 3.) Kill contemplation.

Preserve the Fuel

Discipline works on a fuel system, and everyone's fuel tank is a different size. We each start out our day with a full tank and throughout the course of the day our fuel is used until our tanks are empty. Each decision we make drains a little more of the supply. The fuel is replenished when we sleep and when we wake up we are at full capacity. If you are looking to break a nasty habit, one technique is to preserve the fuel (discipline) for the difficult decisions ahead of you.

I have applied this technique to break several habits. I have used it when dieting and I have used it to quit drinking alcohol. I am a very habitual person by nature. If I do something one time and enjoy it, it takes a lot of discipline for me to remove it from my life. I am very good at deciding which habits to let into my life and which to keep, but drinking was one that began to get out of control.

I am sure a lot of people can relate. Back when I would drink alcohol each day, I would put in a full day's work and then allow myself to drink for just one hour before bed. I enjoyed grabbing some wine, catching up on text messages, and giving my brain a chance to relax.

However, it got to the point where one hour of drinking turned into two. Soon, the habit of relaxing with a glass of wine began to take priority. I started to drop my tasks for the day so I could relax with wine. Drinking and relaxing became the priority and I noticed I was far less productive throughout the week. It was during that time that I decided to quit.

I decided to preserve my discipline "fuel" for the moment I would want to drink. I decided to make every other decision in my day as easy as possible so I could focus my energy solely on changing the habit of drinking. At the time, I was also focused on my diet, and it was taking a lot of discipline to ensure I was eating the way I desired. I immediately loosened up on my diet with the understanding I would go back to it after I quit drinking. I would spend the entire day making as many of my decisions as easy as possible, and when "wine time" hit, I had all my fuel available for the decision. As a result, choosing not to drink was easier. Saving my fuel each day for that difficult moment of decision worked. The technique of preserving the fuel works for all habits that take discipline. Do this for just one area at a time so that all of your fuel is preserved for the habit you are trying hardest to break.

If you fail at any point in time while on your journey to breaking a habit, do not be discouraged. Treat the failure as a test to see how quickly you can start the process again. It may sound cheesy but "getting back on the horse" is exactly what we're trying to accomplish. Measure yourself against how long it takes for you to fall off the horse in the first place. And measure yourself against how long it takes you to get back on. There is no sense in crying over spilled milk. Instead, assess the amount of time it takes you to get started again. See failing as an opportunity to begin working toward beating your last winning streak.

Make It a Critical Task

In order to sustain the progress I made each night (in the alcohol example), I adopted a Power List from CEO Andy Frisella. The concept of the Power List is to write down five critical tasks you need to do to make progress in your life for that particular day. They should be such important tasks that by not doing them you will consider the day to have been lost. Naturally, they should be difficult tasks that you are avoiding. It is usually the things we do not want to do that will afford us the most progress. When you accomplish all five tasks, you "win the day." The objective is to see how many days in a row you can win. I have used Andy's Power List for many things in my life, all with great results. It is the tool I used to quit drinking and it is the tool I have used to build wealth. I am a firm believer in the Power List and establishing critical tasks. As you continue through this book and get to the workout program, I challenge you to make all of your workouts a critical task. It will help you build your discipline and cause you to get in incredible shape.

If you are interested in learning more about Andy Frisella's Power List, he has a podcast called *The MFCEO* where he talks about it frequently. It is a fantastic podcast for those who want to make changes in their lives, whether personal or professional.

Kill Contemplation

The next technique to master discipline is immediate decision making. I kill contemplation with "the Five Second Rule." Our brains have the ability to talk us out of anything; if we give it the time and opportunity to do so. I adapted Mel Robbins' Five Second Rule (discussed earlier) to dismiss any idea of negotiation with myself. I use it to practice making pre-determined decisions within five seconds and to shut out contemplation.

For instance, if you are trying to wake up without hitting your snooze button, count in your head to five when the alarm goes off, and before you finish counting, put your feet to the ground. Your brain will not be able to convince you to stay in bed. The Five Second Rule will allow you to take full control of your actions. You can use the Five Second Rule for any decision you want to be a non-negotiable. Try practicing it in the workout program of this book. On the days you do not feel like working out, decide ahead of time it will not be a choice. When the decision presents itself, use the rule to take action.

Once you master the Five Second Rule within the program, try it in other areas of your life. Stick to only one decision you're struggling with at a time. Sustain the new habit of acting and ruling out contemplation for a 66-day period. Why 66 days? Malcolm Gladwell, author of *Outliers*, states it take 66 consecutive days to lock in a habit. By the 67th day, you will have mastered the ability to rule out contemplation and increased your levels of discipline.

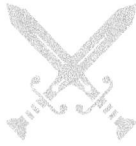

SPECIFICITY

"Your focus determines your reality."
~ George Lucas

The last step in training the mind is to develop the ability to think extremely specifically. In this chapter, I will explain the importance of specificity and how to use it to elevate you to a higher level of performance. Then, in the next chapter, I will give you practical exercises to help you get more specific in your goals.

Much like cutting a diamond, specificity helps to concentrate energy into laser-sharp focus to achieve our goals. The more specific we are about what we want to achieve, the more likely we are to achieve them. For example, making the goal: "to get in better shape" is vague. It is not measurable and therefore unattainable. A better (more specific) goal is: "I want to weigh 190 pounds at six percent body fat." The second goal is very specific and is undeniably measurable.

Consider the importance of specificity versus vagueness while planning for combat. If I gather up the men in my company — soldiers I fight alongside— and tell them the mission is "to figure it out as we go," we will be met with chaos on the objective. There will be confusion about who the enemy is and what friendly forces should do when they encounter them. You can imagine the havoc going into combat without specificity could cause.

In contrast, if I brief a very specific image of the outcome for the mission, we will be much more likely to achieve success. The soldiers will have a very detailed understanding of what is supposed to happen by the end of the mission and there will be clarity on the objective. Soldiers will act deliberately and with certainty to achieve the desired outcome. They will know the details of how to act when they meet the enemy. The soldiers will know what specific actions to take through the end of the mission.

There is such a thing as being overly specific. If I command a soldier to breach a specific door, in a specific way, and leave no other option for him to deal with contingencies, I am setting both the soldier and the organization up for failure. Life follows the same rules.

We have to accept room to react and "develop the situation" in order to achieve the desired outcome. In the book *Team of Teams*, General Stanley McChrystal beautifully demonstrates the idea of adapting to the situation as being "resilient." He describes resiliency as the result of linking elements that allow them to reconfigure in response to change. Resiliency, when coupled with specificity, is an effective way to achieve your goals. Being specific will keep you focused on what you want to achieve. Being resilient will allow you to adapt to changes and modify the plan.

One of my favorite ways to apply specificity is to imagine my ideal future self in great detail. I did this during my training for the 75th Ranger Regiment and I believe it helped me achieve success.

Several months out from selection, I started to imagine what it would feel like if I had achieved my goal of becoming a Ranger. I developed a crystal-clear image of the outcome. I pictured how I would think and feel if I were accepted. I would think about how I would walk, how I would talk, and how I would carry myself if I accomplished my goal. As I mentioned in the visualization section of this book, I rehearsed the image I had for myself daily. Before I went to bed every night, I would visualize it in such detail that I was overwhelmed with the feeling of success.

By compounding this practice each day, I noticed I began to train more intensely. I also noticed I was more likely to think empowering thoughts instead of disempowering ones when I reached fatigue. Additionally, my inner voice would encourage me during times of difficulty. I noticed I was less likely to become discouraged that I would not make it. Through repeated practice of focusing on the specific outcome of becoming a Ranger, every workout made me feel more deserving of becoming one. I started carrying a subtle confidence about me. The feeling of confidence reassured me I would make it. Now, the feeling was not constant, but it helped keep me focused. From time to time I had my doubts; however, the spikes of reassurance kept me focused on my goal when I would otherwise be discouraged. Months after rehearsing the specific image I had of my future self, I was accepted into the 75th Ranger Regiment.

Luckily, the ability to think specifically is skill. It is one we start developing at an early age. When we are kids, we tend to be very specific about who we want to grow up to be. Our need for identity causes us to contemplate who we want to become. We contemplate with whom we should hang out, what clothes we should wear, and what sports to play. Over time, those thoughts turn into actions, and we soon resemble the image we created for ourselves.

I have noticed that as we grow older, people lose sight of the fact we can be specific about who we want to become. Perhaps a child is born before we are ready. Or some unexpected occurrence that requires all of our attention presents itself. People become forced to deal with the various distractions around us and inventing ourselves becomes lost. The specific image of who we want to become fades, and we slowly become products of our environment instead of creators of our reality.

As you continue to progress through this program, adopt the mindset that we all have the ability to change who we are. We all have the same ability to mold our identity to fit our goals. The next chapter will give you a few tools to use to get more specific about your future self. These tools will help you become more deliberate in your fitness goals and encourage you to gain specificity in all that you do.

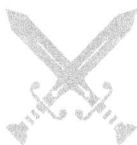

THE WHOLE MAN CONCEPT

"Most people are walking generalities."
~ Ed Mylett

I n order to get specific about what I want in life, I use two exercises. The first is a model I call "The Whole Man *Concept*" and the second is my mission statement. Years ago, I became overwhelmingly frustrated at the life I was living and told myself I had had enough. I told myself I was going to stop limiting what I thought I was capable of and commit myself to achieving my dreams. I told myself I needed to address every area in my life. I created eight dimensions that I believe make up a balanced and complete person. I then assessed myself in each of the areas. I drew the dimensions in a pie chart and drew each one in symmetry with the next. I called it "The Whole Man Concept." I listed what I wanted in each dimension for the short and long term. When I reached the fitness dimension, I began listing all of the personal and professional fitness goals I wanted to achieve. Identifying the fitness goals I wanted to achieve led me to create the workout program you are about to start.

Start a journal or grab a piece of blank paper. I will take you through how to set goals and assess yourself within The Whole Man Concept. These exercises will help you achieve clarity in life and project you to new heights.

The Whole Man Concept

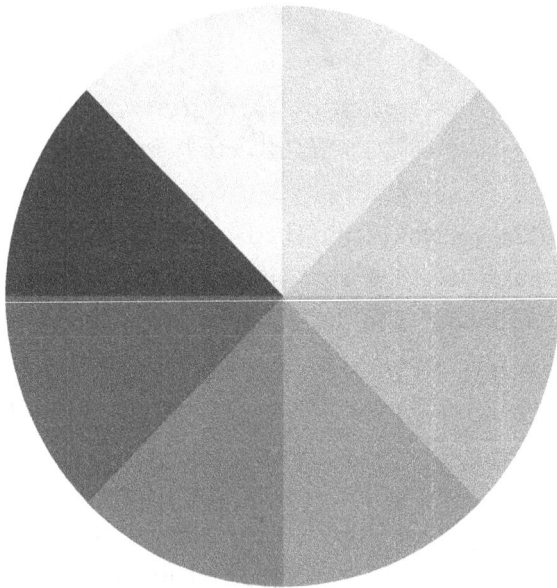

● Materialism ○ Epicureanism ○ Fitness ○ Finances
○ Spirituality ● Relationships ● Profession ● Wisdom

Exercise 1A: List the criteria you believe make up each aspect of a balanced and fulfilled person (The Whole Man).

The list below contains the dimensions that make up The Whole Man, the aspects of which are in **boldface**. For each aspect of the concept, I have added *my own* definition of the term. For example, the *Fitness* dimension for me is about achieving goals that ensure life *Longevity* and *Competition*. The Whole Man Concept dimensions are relative to the individual, meaning each one is defined by the individual. For example, *Spirituality* means different things to different people. For me, being spiritually balanced means meditating once a day and expressing gratitude once a day. Doing that fulfills my sense of spirituality. Use the below model as a guide to create *your own list*.

Complete **Exercise 1A** by listing out the aspects you believe make up a balanced person.

The Whole Man Dimension and Definitions (**my dimensions and definitions**):

1. **Fitness**: Longevity + Competition

2. **Finances**: Financial Freedom

3. **Spirituality**: Gratitude + Relationship with Higher Power

4. **Relationships**: Love + Compassion

5. **Profession**: Fulfillment + Serving a Higher Purpose

6. **Wisdom**: Mental Growth

7. **Materialism**: Pleasure Through Purchase

8. **Epicureanism**: Living and Experiences

Exercise 1A: The Whole Man Dimension and Definitions (**your dimensions and definitions**):

1.

2.

3.

4.

5.

6.

7.

8.

Exercise 1B: Describe what being balanced in each of the eight areas looks like. Consider them on a day-to-day basis, and over the course of life.

_____

_____

_____

_____

_____

_____

_____

_____

_____

_____

_____

Exercise 1C: Write one or more goal you would like to achieve in each of the eight areas you identified as making up a balanced person. Include WHY you chose the goal.

_____

_____

_____

_____

_____

_____

_____

_____

_____

_____

_____

_____

Exercise 2A: Create a Mission Statement for your life. In this exercise, you will create clarity by getting specific about what you want out of life.

Write a short paragraph reflecting on your life as if you have achieved its full potential. This will be your new mission statement. Start the paragraph with the words "By the end of my life, I will have...." My mission statement is below:

"By the end of my life, I will have stories to tell. I will have seen the world, changed countless people's lives, and sought after every opportunity linked to happiness with zero financial barriers and limitations. I will have expressed love toward my friends and family daily, cherished my wife, built unbreakable relationships, and raised remarkable children. I will have expressed gratitude religiously, lived for helping others, and dominated life on my terms."

Now write yours:

_____

_____

_____

_____

_____

Exercise 2B: Create a Personal Motto for your life. For this exercise, write a short phrase that summarizes your approach to how to live each day. In general, the motto should be a few short words or a short sentence. Make it inspiring for you. You will live by this motto for the rest of the program. As a guide, mine is "Dominate Life." Now, write yours:

_____

_____

_____

_____

_____

_____

_____

_____

_____

_____

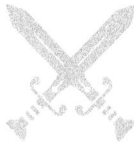

SELF-AWARENESS AND GOAL SETTING

The following exercises will help your increase self-awareness and establish goals in each of the dimensions in The Whole Man Concept.

Exercise 3A: Assess how balanced you are in each of the dimensions of the "The Whole Man" you previously defined.

Draw your own (on a separate piece of paper) or fill in the pie chart to the bottom right of the page. Depict how balanced you are in each area of The Whole Man as you see yourself today. For example, a perfectly balanced person would have eight equal slices of pie within their chart. Keep this chart for yourself; do not let anyone see it. The pie chart is for self-assessment without any influence. If you show someone, your subconscious may alter your decisions. I recommend putting it as the first page in a new journal, as you will reflect on it often. Reference the criteria you listed in Exercise 1A for what each area looks like in a balanced person.

The Whole Man Dimension and Definitions (**your dimensions and definitions**):

1.

2.

3.

4.

5.

6.

7.

8.

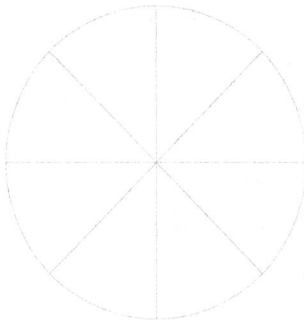

Exercise 3B: Review your Mission Statement and create one short-term goal (weeks or months) and one long-term goal (over one year) per Whole Man Concept dimension you created. Think BIG with all of them — do not hold back.

E.g. Dimension: Fitness
Short-Term Goal: Gain 10 lbs. of muscle in 6 months
Long-Term Goal: Weigh 190 lbs. at 6% body fat in 12 months

1. *Dimension:*	*Short-Term Goal:*
	Long-Term Goal:
2. *Dimension:*	*Short-Term Goal:*
	Long-Term Goal:
3. *Dimension:*	*Short-Term Goal:*
	Long-Term Goal:
4. *Dimension:*	*Short-Term Goal:*
	Long-Term Goal:
5. *Dimension:*	*Short Term Goal:*
	Long Term Goal:
6. *Dimension:*	*Short-Term Goal:*
	Long-Term Goal:
7. *Dimension:*	*Short-Term Goal:*
	Long-Term Goal:

8. Dimension:	Short-Term Goal:
	Long-Term Goal:

Exercise 3C: List out the <u>smallest</u> action you can take to accomplish your short-term goals within each category.

E.g. Dimension: Fitness
Short-Term Goal: Gain 10 lbs. of muscle in 6 months
Actions: Track Fats, Carbs, Protein for 7 days

1. Dimension:	*Short-Term Goal:*
	Action:
2. Dimension:	*Short-Term Goal:*
	Action:
3. Dimension:	*Short-Term Goal:*
	Action:
4. Dimension:	*Short-Term Goal:*
	Action:
5. Dimension:	*Short Term Goal:*
	Action:
6. Dimension:	*Short-Term Goal:*
	Action:
7. Dimension:	*Short-Term Goal:*
	Action:
8. Dimension:	*Short-Term Goal:*
	Action:

Exercise 3D: For each Whole Man dimension, write out how it is going to make you feel to accomplish each of your goals. Then, write out how it is going to make you feel to NOT accomplish it.

Dimension: *Fitness*
Short-term goal: *Gain 10 lbs. of muscle in 6 months*
Long-term goal: *Weigh l 90 lbs. at 6% body fat in 12 months*
Accomplishing my goal will make me feel: *Confident. Powerful. Excited. Rewarded. Accomplished. Deserving. Like a winner.*
Not accomplishing my goal will make me feel: *Horrible. Like a failure. Second class. Unsuccessful. Like a quitter.*

Dimension:
Short-term goal:
Long-term goal:
Accomplishing my goal will make me feel:
Not accomplishing my goal will make me feel:

Dimension:

Short-term goal:

Long-term goal:

Accomplishing my goal will make me feel:

Not accomplishing my goal will make me feel:

Dimension:

Short-term goal:

Long-term goal:

Accomplishing my goal will make me feel:

Not accomplishing my goal will make me feel:

Dimension:

Short-term goal:

Long-term goal:

Accomplishing my goal will make me feel:

Not accomplishing my goal will make me feel:

Dimension:

Short-term goal:

Long-term goal:

Accomplishing my goal will make me feel:

Not accomplishing my goal will make me feel:

THE WHOLE MAN PROJECT

Dimension:

Short-term goal:

Long-term goal:

Accomplishing my goal will make me feel:

Not accomplishing my goal will make me feel:

Dimension:

Short-term goal:

Long-term goal:

Accomplishing my goal will make me feel:

Not accomplishing my goal will make me feel:

SECTION TWO
THE BODY

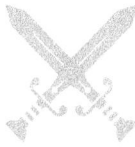

YOU ARE A PROFESSIONAL ATHLETE

O ver the next 12 weeks, adopt the mindset of a professional athlete. A professional puts in the time to master their craft, and is committed to excellence and their highest self. Treat training your body and mind like a profession, not a job. A job implies it is OK to do the bare minimum, and all jobs eventually end, whereas a profession implies going above and beyond, mastering the craft. Professions endure and they are built around striving to achieve excellence.

In order to grow mentally, physically, and spiritually, treat every workout as an opportunity to prepare for battle. Every day you step into training is an opportunity to sharpen your knife for war. Remember, what we do in one area of our life we do in all; therefore, apply your best self to this program. Doing so will create a ripple effect in the other areas of your life. Once you commit to treating fitness as a profession and not a job, you will unlock the ability to reach your highest potential. It is through potential that you will get paid with abundance. Your "payment" will be quality of life, longevity, and CONFIDENCE.

At the end of the day, you are COMPETING against yourself, and you are there to WIN. Not by a little bit. You are not there to just skate by. You are there to dominate. To run the score up as high as you can against your old self. For the next 12 weeks, pay attention to the details of your actions, practice self-study, and challenge yourself. Your capability in the past has no bearing on your future capacity. What matters is that you beat who you are today, again and again. Speak growth in your life and train the body as an outlet to manifest it.

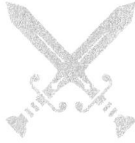

UNDERSTANDING THE WORKOUT PROGRAM

"Collect the dots and then connect the dots."
~ Pete Blaber

The above quote implies problem solving after gathering information. That is precisely how I intend for you to use this program. The program was designed to assist you in seeing "the bigger picture." I wrote it to create BALANCED and FIT athletes. It includes running, weightlifting, Olympic lifting, and rucking. This plan has consistently created athletes who are faster, stronger and smarter than they were before they started.

One individual added 30 lbs. to his squat in eight weeks. Others increased their bench by 20 lbs. or more. Everyone I have trained with this program has gotten faster. Of note, 10 out of 21 officers who used this program in MCCC broke their all-time personal records on their 12-mile ruck march. The one missing ingredient in this program is my personal, one-on-one instruction. To solve that problem, I offer a personalized consultation. Additionally, I am putting together a video series to supplement the program. If you are interested in receiving coaching from me or these videos, my contact information is at the end of the book.

Each day in the program has a purpose. Take the purpose and apply it to the workout and your day. For instance, Monday will read "The purpose of Monday is to SWITCH IT ON." When working out, it is up to you to adopt that mindset for the training session, then tackle everything else with the same mentality. Ideally, you should begin each day by working out so you can set a precedent for the day ahead.

Likewise, each week has a mindset lesson for you to instill and grow your mind. The mindset lessons are the cornerstones of my personal growth. For example, Week 1 is: "Be 1% Better." Each day that week, adopt that mentality. Attack each workout with the intention of being just 1% better. You will also notice that you will start treating other things in your life the same way.

Applying the purpose and the mindset lessons will drastically increase your quality of life; by the end of the week, you will be proud that you not only trained your body, but you trained your mind. Understand that this was written for intermediate athletes, but it is appropriate athletes of all levels. At any point you can scale the workouts back or increase the difficulty of the workouts to meet your individual abilities. If you are a new to fitness, cut each workout in half. If you are an elite athlete, increase the intensity and add additional reps or sets. Cut your rest periods back for the runs and scale the difficulty according to your tolerance.

The running portion was written for individuals who run at least 10 miles total in a week or can complete five miles in one session without issue or injury. All of the weight training is designed for people who are currently working out three to five days a week or have a background in some sport (even if it's been over 10 years). Each week will start with a unit of instruction. It will cover the mindset lesson for the week and any special instructions necessary to ensure the week is executed to its full potential. The overall focus of the entire program is proper form and body mechanics.

The format of the workout program is the most important piece of the entire training approach. It is the best way I have found to concurrently train for cardio, strength, and muscular endurance. The program is meant to be executed from the top and down. It easy to read and easy to follow. Read each workout the day prior and you will be set up for success.

The instruction row across the bottom of the program is used to teach and develop you as an athlete. It includes the classes I teach when I am personally training military athletes. Some days include classes on running. Other days are about lifting. Since I cannot physically be there to coach you, it is up to you to research the instruction for the day. I have written the instruction in terms that are easy to understand with five to 10 minutes of YouTube video searches. Even if you are 100% comfortable with the workout, make a practice of looking up the instruction for the day. On Sundays, there will be tasks for you to study. As the program progresses, the prompts become more vague. As the program becomes less prescriptive, it is up to you continue self-study.

Finally, most training days are designed to take one and a half to two hours to complete. If you go over on time, it is likely you are not attacking the workouts deliberately enough. If your schedule does not accommodate the time necessary to complete the workout at least "check the block" in each event. For example, if you only have one minute left in your day to complete the workout, then do one minute worth of the workout.

Creating great routines and habits are a part of this program. It is important that you go through the entire process each day to assimilate them. Creating habits is the most important part of the program. With great habits, you will continue to reach higher levels of performance even when you are done with the program. Enjoy the journey.

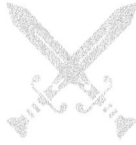

CARDIO: GIVE IT A PURPOSE

"Deliberate practice is purposeful, whereas practice is meaningless."
~ Jeramiah Solven

The first workout of each day is cardiovascular exercise. Typically, you will run three days a week, with an emphasis on intervals. Intervals give you the ability to do more with less. By increasing the intensity, you get more out of your workout, using less time. I have dedicated Monday to Time Trials and Volume Runs, which include distances typically between three and five miles. Wednesday is for Medium Intervals (800m-1200m) and Fridays are a combination of Short Intervals (200m-400m) and Rucking. I use Tuesdays and Thursdays as recovery cardio days. If you are an elite runner, these are great days to accumulate more running volume at a low intensity. For everyone else, Tuesday's and

Thursday's cardio is built to get the heart rate elevated to around 120 bpm and to circulate blood and enable recovery.

Time Trials. Time Trials are built to assess you. You should complete these days at maximum effort and assess yourself. Keep track of your times because you will need them to calculate future paces.

Volume Runs. Time- or distance-based runs intended to accumulate running volume. These are medium-intensity runs, where the heart rate remains around 160 bpm. As a rule of thumb, you should be able to talk during any run where the max heart rate is 160 bpm. Volume days are usually on Monday. Pay attention to the heart rate zone or time allotment dictated for each workout.

Medium Intervals. Target VO2 (volume of oxygen exchanged). They are also used to develop your goal pace for the five-mile race. The intent on these days is to test the threshold of your VO2 Max, allow recovery, then repeat the process while accumulating mileage. The program is built to scale into accumulating five miles of medium intervals. On Medium Interval days, use your goal pace for the five-mile race to calculate the time for each interval. For example, if you are trying to run a 30-minute five-mile, your pace for 800 meters would be three minutes.

Short Intervals. Train for pace only. These are usually less stressful from a cardiovascular standpoint. Make sure to stay disciplined and match your goal pace for every interval.

During all short interval work, focus on body mechanics, economy of running, and pace for the two-mile race. On Short Interval days, use your goal pace for the two-mile race to calculate the time for each interval. For example, if your goal is to run a 12-minute two-mile, then your 400-meter pace would be 90 seconds.

Rucking. I approach rucking with two methods: speed and volume. On the Speed Days, the focus is running with a ruck. Yes, I said it: if you want to get fast with a ruck you have to run with one. A lot of people shun this idea, but if you do it correctly, you can get very fast with a ruck, and do so without injury. To prevent injury, keep a short stride, create momentum by leaning forward with your body, and alternate Speed Days with Volume Days.

Speed Days. On Speed Days, you will see a 3:00/3:00 on technique. What this means is that you will jog for 3:00 and walk for 3:00 for the amount of time specified. On the Volume Days, you will do Forced Rucking. In the Army Infantry, the standard for the 12-mile ruck is to complete it in three hours, which amounts to a 15-minute-a-mile pace.

Forced Ruck. On Forced Ruck days, your pace should be fast enough that it takes effort to maintain the pace, and should not fall below 15 minutes per mile. The Forced Ruck days are nested with the Short Interval days for a reason. Short Interval days do not take very long, and when you couple them with rucking, your body builds up durability quickly. You will need a pair of tennis shoes and boots for Friday. You will use running shoes for the short intervals then boots for the ruck marches. Limit yourself to five to 10 minutes to transition from one to the next.

If rucking is not one of your goals, you can replace it with a different "sport" of your choice. Almost all of the rucking workouts can be converted into swimming or biking workouts. Just follow the format and train yourself according to the prescribed time or intent. If you notice yourself developing physical agitations while rucking, alternate sport workouts are encouraged.

Calculating Pace

The cardio program is written using percentages to dictate pace. To calculate it, take your race pace (in seconds) and divide it by the percentage dictated by each workout.

For example, if your last three-mile race pace was 18:00, then you ran a 6:00/mile pace. If the workout says to run three miles at 90% (of your race pace) then you would run it at a 6:40 pace. See the below example calculation:

Step 1.) 6:00 per mile Race Pace = 360 seconds

Step 2.) 90% Race Pace = 360 (time) ÷ .90 = 400 seconds

Step 3.) 400 Seconds = 6:40 min/mile

90% Race Pace = 6:40 min/mile

Another measure of assessing your pace is to use Rate of Perceived Exertion or RPE. The RPE Chart is a scale from

THE WHOLE MAN PROJECT

1-10 with 10 being max effort. It is based on how much effort you think you are giving. If the workout states to run three miles at 90% race pace, then you would run at a RPE of 9. When using the RPE scale for your workouts, match the percentage prescribed to the chart below.

	RPE Chart
	Rate of Perceived Exertion
10	**Max Effort Activity** Feels almost impossible to keep going Completely out of breath, unable to talk
9	**Very Hard Activity** Very difficult to maintain exercise intensity Can barely breathe, difficult to speak a single word
7-8	**Vigorous Activity** On the verge of becoming uncomfortable Short of breath, can speak a sentence
4-6	**Moderate Activity** Feels like you can exercise for hours Breathing heavily, can hold a short conversation
2-3	**Light Activity** Feels like you can maintain for hours Easy to breathe, can carry on a conversation
1	**Very Light Activity** Anything other than sleeping, watching TV, riding in a car, etc.

Mindset Tool

One thing I like to do when I run is to create a "mental focal point." I give myself a singular thing to think about during the workout. It can be related to body mechanics or a specific goal. I keep my focus on body mechanics on interval days and think of life goals during longer distances. For example, if I am choosing to focus on form, I will pick a lesson to practice like arm swing, and I will practice arm swing for the entire interval.

I will use goals as "mental focal points" as well. During longer runs, I will picture a goal and imagine myself attaining it for the duration of the run. I will replay achieving the goal over and over. Running can be about more than running. It is an opportunity to mentally rehearse your achievements. You get to choose what you focus on; therefore, make sure you choose thoughts that serve you.

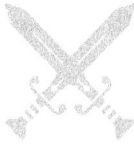

ON RUNNING

"You can teach an old dog a new trick,
and this old dog wants to learn."
~ Thomas P. O'Neil

When I was new to the military, the two-mile run for the Army Physical Fitness Test was something I dreaded. It might as well have been 100 miles. The thought of running an "entire" two miles was exhausting; however, as I began to learn more about running, I slowly removed the mental limitations I had toward it.

It has taken me a long time to become decent at running. By constantly studying and practicing the skill of running, I have continued to improve my running over the course of the past 10 years. As a result, I have gotten in good enough shape to be able to run an unplanned marathon at a moment's notice. I proved it a couple months ago after a friend invited me to one with a day's notice.

Learning how to run more efficiently and developing a running progression will help you achieve unprecedented running heights. I am going to give you the tools I have used to increase my weekly mileage more than five times the amount I use to run. Before I started working on running, I would accumulate around five to 10 miles per week. In contrast, I accumulated 33 miles of running last week. Seven of them were in body armor. Concurrently, I have been able to increase my mileage and stay strong. I have still been able to sustain increases on my squat, deadlift, and military press. By studying the tools in this program, I have been able to accomplish a two-mile time of 11:57 and a five-mile time of 32:33.

Getting better at running has the additional benefit of helping you get better at rucking. I used to struggle with the 12-mile ruck march (completed carrying 35-45lbs). When I first attempted it as a private, my finishing time was just under 4 hours (20-minute miles). Then I started obsessing over running techniques and workouts. From then on, my fitness completely changed. By concentrating my workouts on running, I was able to complete the 12-mile ruck in 1 hour 57 minutes. It is my goal to help reconstruct the way you approach cardio so that you experience the same results.

There are people faster than me, but my progress is impressive. My progress has been a result of working harder and smarter. In the next chapter, I am going to provide some tips and tricks I used to transform my running ability. I have taught these techniques to countless people, and they have always proven effective.

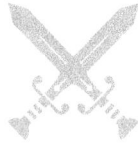

RUNNING FORM

*"The mind is the source of all suffering, but
it is also the source of all happiness."*
~ Pema Chodron

I have a deep belief that most people hate running because they have developed a negative attitude toward it. I believe most people who hate running have a pattern of finishing their runs with a negative experience. You can, however, change that experience.

If you want to start enjoying running, then your last memory from a run should be rewarding. Even if the run is painful, you should finish and mentally "pat yourself on the back" to positively reinforce the experience. Finishing a run positively will make you more likely to run again in the future. It will have a compounding effect and over time you will get in better shape.

One way to make the run enjoyable is to focus more on form and less on effort. At this point, a lot of people reading this might be thinking, "Oh well, I have been running 'my' way for years; it is impossible for me to change." The fact of the matter is I am not teaching an old dog a new trick; we are just refining the old one. Each day you run in this program, focus on making micro alterations to your running form. By learning to run more efficiently, your energy output will decrease and running will become easier. As a result, you will get faster.

Another way to become more efficient at running is to generate all of your energy into one singular direction: forward. Your head should be level to the ground, with your eyes on the horizon, and your chin just slightly down. A lot of people make the mistake of raising their chin while they run. Raising the chin tells your body to lean backward and prevents forward momentum. To generate forward momentum drop the chin a half-inch to an inch from the level position. Your shoulders should be pulled back and not shrugged forward. The arms should form a relaxed 90 degrees and the hands should softly touch the sides of your hips when they swing.

A common mistake with the arm swing is torque. Your arms should move in a linear direction and not across your body. Crossing the body with your arm swing will cause resistance in respiration and make breathing more difficult. Imagine you are holding a potato chip in each of your hands when you run. You want the potato chip to stay intact, and you want to brush it against the side of your hips as you are running. Your hands should be nice and loose to prevent the chip from breaking.

Your stomach should be slightly concave and not overly extended. A relaxed stomach will make respiration easier, and you will create a more natural body lean. Use your hips to help set your speed. The further you push them forward, the faster you will naturally want to go. A proper body lean is approximately 15 degrees starting at your ankles. Use the hips to put your body into that position. I like to think of the body lean like a man on a unicycle. If he starts to lean forward, he begins to move forward. The same applies to your body mechanics.

To reduce the amount of energy it takes to project you forward, dial in the body lean and the turnover of your legs. Much like pedaling a bike, the turnover is the rotation of your legs, which generates movement. Engage your hamstrings to generate the turnover. A common mistake is people assume the quadriceps are primarily responsible for the turnover; however, the role of the quadriceps is leg extension. The hamstrings are responsible for the rate at which your legs turn. They are responsible for your speed. The hamstrings should do approximately 75% of the work.

Another common mistake when running is overextending your legs. When I was enlisted, it was common to hear people yell at soldiers to "stride it out" when trying to get them up to speed. This is horrible advice. Overextending your legs causes "breaking."

Throwing your leg out in front of your midline will slow you down and prevent forward momentum. Instead, shorten your stride so that your turnover almost feels choppy and increase the rate of your leg rotation. Run with your head over your feet. To check your stride, look down at your lower leg, and make sure your entire shin is not exposed as you extend your leg forward. If you can see the entire shin, it is likely that you are overextending and breaking. To correct it, shorten your stride and speed up your turnover. Bring the front knee high so that it is parallel with the ground before you strike the ground. The turnover should mirror riding a bike. Emulate the way you would pedal and put the emphasis in the turnover.

In regard to the foot strike, I personally prefer a midfoot strike because it is the most natural. If you watch somebody run barefooted, they will land with the front pad of their foot first and their heel second. A midfoot strike is biomechanically efficient. It allows for proper activation of the ankle. Our ankles are meant to help absorb the shock of running. Landing with a midfoot strike helps disperse the impact through the ankle and lower extremity.

To practice the midfoot strike, try barefoot running on a soft surface. Jog short distances of 50-100 meters to become more aware of how your body naturally comes into contact with the ground. Then replicate the strike with shoes on. To achieve a proper midfoot strike, you will have to wear a shoe conducive to it. I personally enjoy a "zero drop" shoe.

A zero-drop shoe is one without a slope to bottom of the shoe. If you are going to adopt a new shoe to go along with a new foot strike, I recommend you do it gradually to prevent injury. Start with shorter distances and keep yourself injury-free. Drastic changes can lead to quick injuries. Be cautious, but do not be afraid to experiment.

If you want more information on running form, I recommend researching the POSE Method. It is a technique that has helped me significantly. I have used it to set numerous personal records. I have even used the POSE Method to help others break theirs. I trained a guy who struggled for years to break a 12:30 two-mile. After two months of coaching we shaved his two-mile run from a 13:00 to a 12:20, all because I taught him the POSE Method. I believe in it so much that you will see the POSE Method show up as part of your homework in the workout program.

At first, you might feel more exhausted while trying the running methods I have discussed in this chapter. That is because you are learning a new skill. It takes energy and focus to develop good running habits. Stay consistent and patient, and you will begin to lock in the form and run with ease.

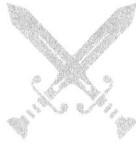

STRENGTH TRAINING

"Ain't nothing but a peanut!"
~ Ronnie Coleman

The main areas of focus for the strength portion of the program are Bench, Squat, and Deadlift. I have implemented some Olympic lifting and compound movements to ensure you (the athlete) get a well-rounded program that exposes weaknesses.

Monday, Tuesday, and Thursday are typically reserved for the aforementioned "big three." On Wednesdays, you will work on pull-ups. Then, on most Fridays, you will focus on full body lifts that challenge multiple anatomical movement planes. There are three movement planes: the frontal, sagittal, and transverse. You will train in each of these planes to help prevent injury and to prevent muscular imbalances.

Most of us are used to working out in one dimension, moving predominantly in one plane. When you train in one plane, you neglect supporting muscle groups, especially under load. For example, runners typically move forward in the sagittal plane, which can cause them to neglect stabilizer muscle groups. Turkish Get-ups are an example of one exercise that puts the body through the transverse and frontal movement planes with weight. Challenging multiple planes provides cross-directional stress on our bodies, and our bodies become more resilient. You can expect to see movements that challenge multiple planes throughout the program; now you know why.

It is always risky to train heavily, especially when introducing new lifts. Therefore, start light and lock in the form throughout this program. Your form at the beginning of the program is the standard. Regardless of your old "high school record," use this program to start from scratch. Be the athlete everybody admires for using appropriate weight. Be the person known for doing the exercises right. Lift intelligently.

I tailored most of the strength workouts to under five reps per set with the intention of increasing the athlete's one-repetition maximum. Progressive overload is used to increase the athlete's strength. You will notice that the program increases by reps some weeks and by sets in others. If an exercise is new for you, then the first step is to establish a 1RM (one-rep max) without any weight. Prove that you can move your body through the lift before increasing the load. It is acceptable to scrutinize your form. Even elite athletes need to go back to the drawing board and start rebuilding their base from scratch. Injuries happen and knowledge fades. Regardless of the skill level, every person going through this program should refresh their knowledge by practicing the appropriate form.

You will learn proper form for all of the lifts by doing the assigned homework each week. I have designed the program so the athlete develops the habit of researching and learning. Each week, you will be given study material to set you up for the week ahead. The "Instruction" row in the workout program will have all the tools you will need to be successful.

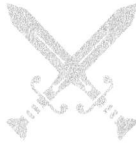

MUSCULAR ENDURANCE TRAINING

"Flow is the optimal level of consciousness… flow follows focus."
~ Steven Kotler

M uscular endurance is the muscles' ability to sustain repeated contractions against a resistance for a period of time. Max push up in two minutes is an example of a muscular endurance test. You will train muscular endurance frequently throughout the week. Each day is designed to give you an opportunity to train for muscular strength and endurance. Training for both can be difficult and usually comes with a tradeoff; however, I have found most people think that tradeoff occurs a lot sooner than it actually does. It is difficult to be an ultra-marathon runner and a world-class powerlifter. However, it is achievable to increase your bench to over 300 lbs. and run an 18-minute three-mile. The model to which you are about to be exposed is the most effective method I have found to train somebody for strength and endurance in one workout session.

Cardio is a lot of people's "kryptonite." I program it up front to make the athlete "eat the frog" before they can get to the fun stuff. When you get to the lifting portion of each day, the reps and sets are written in the program. Each day has the specified reps and sets written under the day of the week or along the left side of the program. Of note, some of the workouts are not overly descriptive for example, "Chest and Triceps exercises for 30 minutes." This was done intentionally to leave options for the athlete and provide flexibility. Not everyone will have access to a world-class gym when they start this program. It is far more important that the athlete achieves the intent for the day rather than the specific exercise.

The most important part of muscular endurance training is that the athlete approaches it to reach a flow state. Getting "in the zone" will pay dividends. It will ensure the athlete is focused on the effect they are trying to create. I think of this mentality as "Effects Before Reps." The effect the athlete is looking for is muscle failure to increase muscular endurance and hypertrophy. I specifically used the word "flow" previously because flow is the moment when you perform your best. It is a matter of getting "in the zone." Approach each muscular endurance workout with the intention to get into flow and reach muscle failure. Most people fail during muscular endurance training because they never reach a flow state. Flow can even be applied to non-physical activities like reading. Have you ever picked up a book and it took you a few minutes or pages to get captured by the story, but once it hit, you could not put it down? That is flow — the ability to block out everything and perform your best.

Just like with the cardio portion of the program, feel free to tailor the muscular endurance training to your fitness level. Make adjustments as necessary. The workouts will be as easy or as hard as you make them.

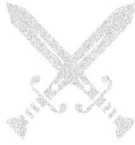

CORE WORK AND INJURY PREVENTION

"Everything you do takes you closer to or further away from your goals."
~ Craig Ballantyne

I designed this program to develop the abdominal muscles for sit-ups, aesthetics, and injury prevention. You will work abs a minimum of three days a week. Tuesday is for sit-up improvement, working the rectus abdominis with upper abdominal concentration. Wednesday is for planks, working external oblique muscles to create a stronger core while improving posture. Thursday is for rectus abdominis with a lower abdominal focus.

The key to core training is short rest periods and keeping the core under constant tension. You will get a lot of core work in some of the muscular endurance workouts doing compound lifts and moving in multiple planes; how-

135

ever, dedicate some time solely to training them by including them at the end of the workout.

Mobility, Foam Rolling, and Flexibility

In the last decade, injury prevention has seen a lot of attention. With so many terms out there, it is important to understand some of the different terminology so that you, as an athlete, can properly apply them to your training regime.

"**Mobility**" is the ability of a joint to move through a range of motion. Increasing mobility can be accomplished through dynamic stretching or foam rolling.

"**Foam rolling**" is a type of self-myofascial release therapy. It removes the adhesions on the fascia to increase elastic on the soft tissue. Foam rolling gives a massage-type feeling and is a great way to address muscle tightness.

"**Flexibility**" is the ability to lengthen the muscle through a range of motions and is often improved through static stretching.

For each of these methods of injury prevention, use a process when you execute them. A routine or system is efficient so you are not wasting time by thinking through what you should do. I like to start from my feet and work my way toward my head for foam rolling.

For mobility training and flexibility, I like to work from the top of the body down. If you are new to mobility training and foam rolling, I highly recommend the book

Supple Leopard by Kelly Starrett. His book is by far the best resource I have come across to teach anyone the basics of mobility training. Additionally, he has a website that offers a free seven-day trial at www.mobilitywod.com, where you can research and look up specific mobility exercises for areas in your body where you have agitations or tightness.

Another great website is www.romwod.com, which has guided videos to teach the viewer how to properly stretch. There are tons of foam rolling YouTube videos that give great demonstrations.

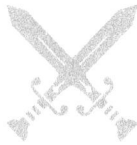

TRAINING MINDSET

"Infuse heart, soul, spirit, and passion
because talent is not enough."
~ Dominick Cruz

Every day you step into a workout, you are going to approach it with a singular objective: training the body and mind. This 12-week program gives you the tools you will need to train both concurrently. Every week, a new mindset focus will be mentioned.

Enforce the Mindset

The mindset tools I am giving you will come from some of the material we have already discussed. Some will come from a few new concepts. I will list the mindset objective, and for the entire week you will adopt it into your workout. For example, the mindset lesson in Week One is "Be 1% Better." As you are walking into the gym, adopt the belief that you can and will "Be 1% Better." Treat it as a mantra and think those words repeatedly. As you start warming up, every rep is a way for you to earn that belief. Every rep, every set, is about proving your commitment to incremental growth. Chant the belief in your mind.

As your body's energy becomes elevated, endorphins will be released, and the belief will become powerful and over-whelming. Each rep and interval will feel like you are leveling up with the mantra. It will become a part of you, and it will become believable. You will be able to feel it and visualize it. Step into that moment and live that belief for the entire work-out. After repeating the mantra for the entire workout, you will notice the feeling will compound across your day. It will carry over to other aspects of your life. Soon, you will notice that everything is becoming 1% better — your relationships, your finances, and all of the areas of The Whole Man Concept.

Continue each workout for the remainder of the week with the same mental lesson to instill it as a core belief. Over the course of 12 weeks, review each previous beliefs and con-tinue to compound its effects. By the end of the 12 weeks, you will have 12 core beliefs that will create the new you.

Contingencies

On days where your workout is interrupted or time is cut short, find a way to implement the mindset lesson for the week. If you can only get one sit-up in before an unexpected obligation, DO THE ONE SIT-UP and use it to ENFORCE the mindset lesson.

The purpose of the workouts is to train both the body and mind. The program is designed to give you an actionable outlet to ensure you are acting on those lessons. ACT on the lessons and drive them into your core though repetition.

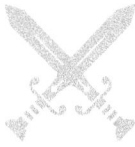

DIET AND NUTRITION

"The chains of habit are too light to be felt
until they are too heavy to be broken."
~ Warren Buffett

The health and fitness industry is saturated with trends, false advertising, and misinformation. More often than not, food is treated like a business. This can make it difficult to know what is and isn't good for you. In order to provide a broad understanding of nutrition, I will give a brief overview of some of the popular diets, then give my approach on how to eat to increase performance. The following is a summary of well-known diets:

The Ketogenic Diet: A fat- and protein-based diet that focuses on using fats for energy over carbohydrates.

The Paleo Diet: Based on foods eaten by early humans. Meals consist of veggies, meats, and fruit. The rule for paleo is "if a caveman did not eat it, you shouldn't either."

Vegetarian: Consumption of non-animal-based foods, with or without dairy products.

Vegan: Excludes meats, eggs, and dairy, as well as all other animal-derived ingredients.

The Mediterranean Diet: Characterized by a high consumption of plant-based foods like whole grains, legumes, nuts, and vegetables.

A Raw Diet: Based on eating foods that are uncooked or unprocessed.

Low-Carb: Usually limits carbohydrates to around 50 grams a day.

A No-Sugar Diet: Avoiding foods with sugar in them, including fruit.

The Macro-based Diet: Based on consuming a measured amount of proteins, fats, and carbs. This is known as "flexible dieting" since the premise of the diet is that if you meet your macros, the rest of your diet will fall into place.

Intermittent Fasting: Restricting food intake for a set time period. Allows your body to fully cleanse itself of food and complete the digestion process.

Out of all of these, I enjoy a macro-based diet; however, I routinely practice fasting. I use fasting to practice discipline and reinforce food as a reward and not a right. Additionally, I have read studies where there was a relationship between longevity and people who fast, and I appreciate it for that relationship. Choose your diet based on what is most effective. The most effective approach to dieting is to do what yields you results, not what you prefer, so "think like an inventor" and discover what works and does not work while doing this program.

If you need more help with your diet, there are six steps you can do to generate a great one. They are: 1.) Pay attention to how you feel. 2.) Have simple eating rules. 3.) Experiment with what works and does not work. 4.) Focus your effort on the most negative items. 5.) Adjust your habits. 6.) Change the way you think about food.

1.) Pay attention to how you feel.

Our days should only consist of things that give us energy. Friends, activities, and food are no exception. You should feel good about 15 minutes after you eat, not immediately after. Fast food restaurants have foods that make you feel extremely rewarded after eating, but the food is horrible for you. Give yourself 15 minutes after you eat to assess the food quality. Have you ever eaten a lunch that left you tired and lethargic? Lunch should give us the energy for the second half of the day. If it drains you, modify parts of your meal until you discover what foods give you energy and which pull it from you. Develop the optimal "formula."

When I started assessing how my meals made me feel, I discovered I do better on a lower-carb lunch. Carbohydrates can cause an insulin spike and a crash following consumption. I cut my carb intake in half, and I started focusing on vegetable-based meals.

2.) Have simple rules.

More important than the diet we follow are the simple rules we have that shape our behaviors. Ninety percent of overweight people have poor eating rules. Developing healthy rules will make food decisions easier. Some rules that work well for me are: no microwavable foods, no processed foods, no soda, no candy/sweets (unless I plan the treat into my day).

My eating habits are far from perfect; however, having simple rules has helped me make fast, healthy food decisions. When I abide by my rules and I forget lunch, the first thing I think of is where I can get food that fits my criteria instead of what is convenient. This practice channels my focus in a positive direction and helps me discover foods that are healthy.

3.) Experiment.

Experimenting with diets is healthy. By trying different foods and assessing how you feel afterward, you will discover the foods that make you perform the best. Once you find the foods that give you more energy throughout the day, eat more of them. If the food makes you feel sluggish after you eat it, get rid of it and never eat it again.

Lastly, remove the negative stigma toward any diet you despise and have not tried. In fact, I challenge you to try them. If you are against a vegetarian diet, then give it a shot. By exposing yourself to the foods you normally avoid, you may discover an increase in your physical performance.

There are numerous weightlifters stepping into the vegetarian lifestyle with profound results. Kendrick Farris switched to a vegan diet in 2014 and became an Olympic athlete in 2016. He stated that the diet gave him more energy and allowed him to recover faster. He would never have learned this without experimentation and trial and error.

4.) Focus your effort on the most negative items.

The fourth method to improve your diet is to focus your energy on a few important items that have the most negative effect. Identify the most damaging food in your diet and remove it. Do not focus on changing every single meal that you consume. That takes too much energy and is a waste of time. Instead, make alterations to the way you currently eat and save your discipline for when it matters the most. We talked previously about how discipline works on a fuel tank. Save the fuel in your tank for the moments when you are at your weakest. Focus your energy on that food and say no to the food that is hurting you the most. Refer to the section on discipline for a refresher on how to improve yours.

I learned the method of focusing on the most negative items from a theory called Pareto's Principle. Pareto's Principle states that 20% of what we do yields 80% of our results. I love this theory because it is a more universal law, which can be found all around us. If you consider a lake, 80% of its volume comes from 20% of the streams that flow into it. Another example is in real estate. In a hotel, the most expensive rooms at the highest floors make up 20% of the total rooms but likely yield 80% of the profits for the entire building. As you get higher and higher in the building, you run into the penthouses and suites. Inside of those, 20% makes up 80% profits for that floor. Pareto's Principle will state that the problem with diet comes from 20% of what we routinely eat. So in order to make a change, do not pay attention to the entire diet, put your energy toward the 20% that is destroying you.

5.) Adjust your habits.

The fifth way to drastically improve your diet is by adjusting your habits. Charles Duhigg wrote a fantastic book called *The Power of Habit*, which breaks down how habits are formed and the power they hold. Habits are reinforced at the subconscious level, causing most of our decisions to occur without active thought. In the book, he studied a man named Eugene who had a disease that destroyed his memory. He could not recall where his kitchen was even when he was in his own home. However, scientists discovered Eugene was able to do the walk alone and return home after repeated walks around the block with his wife. He developed the habit of completing the walk at the subconscious level. Eugene could not recall where he was or draw a map of the area, but his body acted on the habits he built. The scientists discovered we can train ourselves to make subconscious decisions by creating habits.

Charles Duhigg breaks down the habit process and says it consists of a three-step loop: the Cue, Routine, and Reward. The "cue" triggers our brain to choose which routine to go into. The "routine" dictates the behavior that follows. The "reward" occurs in a form of positive stimulus that tells your brain to save the routine. To break the habit loop in your brain, start replacing the reward.

For example, if your routine is to grab some greasy deep-fried chicken from your favorite fast-food restaurant on your way home from work, continue to go to the restaurant but change the chicken. You can start with something else that is unhealthy but equally rewarding so that reward is sustained but you have already started forming a new habit. Continue that method and replace the second item with a third and fourth. Next, change the restaurant. Pick a different one and a new food choice. As you start swapping out items on the new routine, replace them with slightly healthier options until you get to the healthiest scenario.

6.) Change the way you think about food.

The sixth way to make drastic improvements in your diet is to change the way you *think* about food. How we think about food determines our health. We can view it as a tool, a reward, or an inconvenience. The choice is ours. I like to view food as a tool and something to reward behavior. I will plan large meals around intense training and create a situation where I am unquestionably deserving of abundance. These meals are not to be confused with "cheat days." I personally do not believe in a cheat day because it creates a bad habit of eating poor foods too often.

The idea of a cheat day has been so overly used that it has turned into a full day of gluttony. A cheat *meal* was created to reward somebody for a lengthy and strict diet over an extended time frame. Imagine carb cycling for two months and giving yourself a stack of pancakes for making it. Well, cheat *meals* evolved into cheat *days*, and now, people are boasting about their cheat days when they have not done anything to deserve them.

Additionally, the whole idea of a routine cheat day is absurd. It is counterproductive and leaves people with poor foods in their body for the majority of the week. People will drink on Friday and Saturday, then eat like garbage on Sunday. On Monday and Tuesday, the food from Sunday is still in their body. They might eat clean on Wednesday and Thursday but before they know it, Friday is here, and the routine starts all over again. Basically, they get two days of eating healthily out of a seven-day week — hardly a healthy lifestyle.

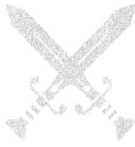

THE BASICS OF SUPPLEMENTS

*"The level of effort you tolerate from
yourself will define your life."*
~ Tom Bilyeu

In this section, I will briefly cover popular supplements. The purpose of this section is to provide you as the reader with a general overview so that you have a basic understanding of what is in the market. Think of this section as a starting point for your future supplement endeavors.

Creatine. One of the most widely studied supplements on the market. Creatine provides the necessary fuel to power the adenosine triphosphate (ATP) process, and naturally occurs in your body. It can be found in foods like beef, chicken, and fish. It is also produced naturally in the liver. The role of creatine is to replenish ATP when the phosphate bonds are broken and used for energy. ATP is used for quick sprints of energy. It is a good supplement to increase power and muscle strength. Supplemental creatine increases the volume of available fuel to power ATP.

Protein (Casein, Whey, Mix, Vegan). Whey and casein protein come from dairy. When processed, they are separated from each other and sold individually. Casein protein is known for being a slower digesting protein and is an acceptable option for meal replacement. Whey protein is a faster digesting protein and is highly recommended immediately following intense weight training. Data shows that your body is at a peak anabolic state within one hour after you train; therefore, supplementing with whey protein is the fastest way to supply the muscle with fuel for growth.

Vegetable proteins come from a variety of sources like peas, brown rice, soy, hemp, chia, and flax. The total protein content varies from each source. One of the most notable combinations is a pea and rice combination protein. Together, they have a high content of essential amino acids and less creatine than some of the other proteins. When comparing, focus on how well your body digests each specific protein. If a dairy-based protein is giving you digestion issues, try switching to a vegetable based source.

Additionally, when selecting a protein, pay attention to how the protein is processed. Because the supplement industry is so large, the quality of products available tends to be poor. Businesses sell their products in a way that gives them bigger margins instead of building a better product. They will process their protein fast and with high temperatures to increase throughput. Doing this diminishes the protein's quality. Look for what is called "Cross Flow Microfiltered Low Temperature Processed" protein for quality product. I personally prefer the supplement company 1st Phorm for protein.

BCAAs (Branch Chain Amino Acids). BCAAs are one of my favorite supplements. They are inexpensive and do wonders for preserving muscle when losing weight. Dieting is a catabolic process and leads to muscle breakdown. As you lose weight, the body pulls from muscle for energy. BCAAs help defend against this process by stimulating protein synthesis and increasing the cell's capacity for protein synthesis. I commonly use BCAAs when conducting military training or missions. BCAAs help me retain strength that would otherwise be lost when conducting extraneous activity. I keep a Ziploc bag of them in my canteen pouch when I road march. Additionally, I will keep a supply on me while on target conducting missions.

Multivitamins. Multivitamins are a great source of minerals. They are the best way to ensure you are not missing vital micronutrients without taking a blood test and monitoring your diet. Multivitamins are especially great for dieting. You are more likely to be missing vital minerals when you are in a caloric deficit. Taking a multivitamin will help increase your energy level and decrease the chance of getting sick.

Fish Oil. Fish oil supplements come from fatty fish. There are numerous health benefits to taking fish oils, which include improved cholesterol levels, liver support, and brain support. One of the key benefits of fish oils is that they can reduce inflammation. Chronic inflammation can hinder athletic performance, so consider supplementing with fish oils to help keep you training by limiting inflammation. Fish oils can help build muscle by regulating cell growth and increasing protein synthesis. Fish oil has also been shown to help regulate the hormones responsible for increasing testosterone levels.

Electrolytes. Electrolytes facilitate rapid electrical impulses across cell membranes and regulate the fluids in the body. They assist with hydration by creating a balance between sodium and potassium within the body's cell membranes. Electrolyte drinks typically consist of sodium (Na+), potassium (K+), calcium (Ca2+), bicarbonate (HCO3-), magnesium (Mg2+), chloride (C1-), and hydrogen phosphate ($HPO4^{2-}$). The symptoms of electrolyte imbalance can include twitching, cramping, and weakness. Drink electrolytes before, during, and/or after cardio. They will help you prevent cramping and keep your body hydrated.

Pre-Workout. Pre-workout is the most commonly purchased type of supplements on the market; however, they typically have the fewest performance enhancing effects. They are less beneficial for the body than other supplements I have covered. Treat pre-workout supplements as a catalyst if you decide to take them. Use them to prime yourself for the gym, but do not rely on them to increase performance. Tailor your pre-workout to the sport you are training for. You will find that more companies are starting to create sport-specific supplements. My recommendation is to research all the ingredients in the supplements you take. With the market always changing, you never know what you could be putting in your body.

SECTION THREE

WORKOUT PROGRAM

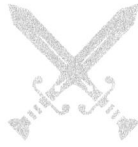

THE WHOLE MAN PROGRAM

Welcome to the workout portion of the book. For the next 12 weeks, every workout is about training the BODY and the MIND. Step into each workout with the intention of training them collectively.

THE MAN IN THE ARENA

It is not the critic who counts;
not the man who points out how the strong man stumbles,
or where the doer of deeds could have done them better.
The credit belongs to the man who is actually in the arena,
whose face is marred by dust and sweat and blood;
who strives valiantly; who errs, who
comes short again and again,
because there is no effort without error and shortcoming;
but who does actually strive to do the deeds;

who knows great enthusiasms, the great devotions;
who spends himself in a worthy cause;
who at the best knows in the end the
triumph of high achievement,
and who at the worst, if he fails, at
least fails while daring greatly,
so that his place shall never be with those cold
and timid souls who neither know victory nor defeat.

– Theodore Roosevelt

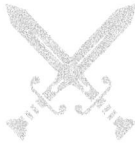

THE TRAINING SPLIT

The next page is the template for the training split you are about to start. It is the framework for the entire program. On the top of the page is a place for you to write the mission statement you wrote during Goal Setting. Along the left side of the training split is the sequence of training. Each week has a specified intensity listed along the top. Use the intensity levels as a guide to gauge your effort during training. On High-Intensity weeks, you should be going 100% on your effort. During Medium Intensity weeks, give 80% effort. The program is written to cycle intensity levels. Rotating the intensity will prevent injuries and allow for the body to adapt to the exercises to maximize performance.

YOUR MISSION STATEMENT

"The Whole Man" Training Split – *Low-, Medium High-Intensity Level*

	Sunday	Monday	Tuesday	Wednesday	Thursday	Friday	Saturday
Purpose	The Purpose of Sunday is to Reset and Refocus in a Capacity THAT WORKS FOR YOU	The Purpose of Monday Is to SWITCH IT ON	The Purpose of Tuesday Is to STACK WINS	The Purpose of Wednesday Is to GENERATE MOMENTUM	The Purpose of Thursday Is to TRY SOMETHING HARD	The Purpose of Friday Is to EARN IT FOR THE WEEKEND	The Purpose of Saturday Is to DO SOMETHING FUN OR NEW
Cardiovascular Endurance	Research POSE Running	Time Trials or Volume Run (3-5 Miles)	15 Minutes Low-impact Cardio (bike/row/walk) Heart Rate: 110-120 bpm	Medium Intervals 800m-1200m Repeats	15 Minutes Low-impact Cardio (bike/row/walk) 110-120 bpm	Short Intervals + Rucking	Light Activity Outside or Something Fun (swimming)
Strength (unless specified) • 6 Sets x 3 Reps at a weight you can complete all 6 sets with	Explore / Research Powerlifter/ Olympic Lifter of Choice (e.g. Dimitry Klokov)	Bench Press (or similar)	Back Squat (or similar)	Pull-ups (Assisted or Unassisted)	Deadlift (or similar)	None	None required

YOUR MISSION STATEMENT

"The Whole Man" Training Split – Low-, Medium High-Intensity Level

	Sunday	Monday	Tuesday	Wednesday	Thursday	Friday	Saturday
Muscular Endurance (unless specified) • **3 exercises per muscle group** • **3-4 Sets x 15-20 Reps for each Exercise** • **30 seconds to 1 minute rest between sets** • **2-3 minutes rest between exercises**	Read or watch a documentary about a successful athlete	Push-up Drill 3 sets MAX push-ups for time or something similar to pre fatigue yourself -Chest/Triceps/Shoulder Exercises for 30 Minutes	Legs – Quad focus for 30 Minutes	Back Biceps for 30 minutes	Legs – Hamstring, Glutes, Lower Back Focus	12- to 18-Minute Circuit Target the full body; kettle bells are a good option. Challenge multiple planes frequently	None Required (touch on any areas of emphasis or do a lift for fun)
Core **For each ab exercise chosen, do 3 sets to failure, rest 30 seconds between sets and 2 minutes between exercises**	N/A	Abdominals 10-15 Minutes Sit-up Improvement Targeting Upper abs	Planks (5-10 Minutes)	Abdominals 10-15 Minutes Sit-up Improvement targeting lower abs; do leg raises/knee raises	Planks (5-10 Minutes)	Abdominals 10-15 minutes targeting oblique muscles	None Required

161

YOUR MISSION STATEMENT

"The Whole Man" Training Split – Low-, Medium- High-Intensity Level

	Sunday	Monday	Tuesday	Wednesday	Thursday	Friday	Saturday
Mobility	N/A	Static Stretching	Foam Roll	Static Stretching	Foam Roll	Static Stretching	None Required
Goal	Self-education	Establish Race Pace	Strength/Conditioning	Pace and VO2 Training	Strength/Conditioning	Pace Training, Volume & Working In Alternate Plane	None Required
Instructions	Recharge Mentally and Physically	Set a Precedent	Compound Your Wins	Acknowledge How Much You Have Changed	Expand What You Know	Test Yourself	Appreciate the Process
Other	Visualization – Visualize Your Future Body, You Achieving Your Goals in Body, Mind, and Spirit. Visualize Perfect Balance and Discipline (10 Minutes)	Meditate for 10 Minutes (download Headspace app for free trial)	Meditate for 10 Minutes (download Headspace app for free trial)	Meditate for 10 Minutes (download Headspace app for free trial)	Meditate for 10 Minutes (download Headspace app for free trial)	Meditate for 10 Minutes (download Headspace app for free trial)	Optional – Practice Visualization

"Dominate LIFE"

What You Do in One Area of Your Life, You Do in All

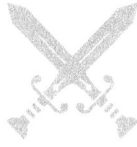

WEEK 1: BE 1% BETTER

<u>Quote:</u> *"The journey of a thousand miles begins with one step."*
~ Lao Tzu

Mission: Week 1s is about establishing your baseline for all the critical tasks we previously identified. Assess your squat, deadlift, bench, five-mile run, 2:00 push-ups, 2:00 sit-ups with perfect form. Approach those events with maximum effort and record your score. For everything else, complete it with medium intensity.

Special Instructions: Get familiar with the entire format of the program. Read over the entire template. Pay special attention to Sunday's tasks. Review all of the instructions row for the entire week. For awareness, the POSE Running Method consists of three phases: Pose, Fall, Pull. Google everything in the instructions row as a refresher.

Mindset for the Week: For the entire week, step into EVERY workout with the mindset of becoming 1% better. Every time something gets tough, repeat that mindset — say it in your head like a mantra. Stack 100 days, and you will be 100% better. Stack that mentality for life.

	Sunday	Monday	Tuesday	Wednesday	Thursday	Friday	Saturday
Purpose	The Purpose of Sunday is to Reset and Refocus in a Capacity THAT WORKS FOR YOU	The Purpose of Monday Is to SWITCH IT ON	The Purpose of Tuesday Is to STACK WINS	The Purpose of Wednesday Is to GENERATE MOMENTUM	The Purpose of Thursday Is to TRY SOMETHING HARD	The Purpose of Friday Is to EARN IT FOR THE WEEKEND	The Purpose of Saturday Is to DO SOMETHING FUN OR NEW
Cardiovascular Endurance	Research POSE Running	5-Mile Individual Assessment Time Trial	15 Minutes Low-impact Cardio (bike/row/walk) Heart Rate at 110-120 bpm	Running Mechanics Drills. Short Interval Repeats at Goal Pace: 10 x 200m w/2:00 rest	15 Minutes Low-impact Cardio (bike/row/walk) Heart Rate at 110-120 bpm	Medium Interval Repeats at Goal Pace: 5 x 800m w/2:30 Rest	Light Activity Outside or Something Fun (swimming, hiking etc..)
Strength (unless specified) • 6 Sets x 3 Reps at a weight you can complete all 6 sets with	Explore/Research Olympic Lifter Dimitry Klokov	None	Squat – Establish 1RM	Establish Max Pull-ups – Pronated grip	Deadlift – Establish 1RM	None	None Required

Table caption: "The Whole Man Program" WEEK 1 (Medium-Intensity Week)

"The Whole Man Program" WEEK 1 (Medium-Intensity Week)	Sunday	Monday	Tuesday	Wednesday	Thursday	Friday	Saturday
Muscular Endurance (unless specified) • 3 Exercises per muscle group • 3-4 Sets x 15-20 Reps for Each Exercise • 30 seconds to 1 minute rest between sets • 2-3 minutes rest between exercises	Read about a successful athlete. E.g. David Goggins, Navy Seal	Max Push-ups in 2:00 Max Sit-ups in 2:00 Chest and Triceps Exercises for 30 Minutes. Superset 2 Exercise for all 30 Minutes	4 Rounds with the same dumbbells: 10 DB Cleans, 50' Lunges, 50' Farmers Carry	Back and Bicep Exercises for 30 Minutes. Superset 2 Exercise for all 30 Minutes	None required	2-5 Rounds: 20 Pistols (10 each leg), 20 Toes to Bar, 30 Push-ups	None Required (touch on any areas of emphasis)
Core For each Ab exercise chosen, do 3 sets to failure, rest 30 seconds between sets and 2 minutes between exercises	N/A	None	15 Minutes Sit-up Improvement Upper Abdominal Focus	Planks: Front, Right, Left, 3 rounds @ 60 seconds	15 Minutes Sit-up Improvement Lower Abdominal Focus	None	None Required

"The Whole Man Program" WEEK 1 (Medium-Intensity Week)

	Sunday	Monday	Tuesday	Wednesday	Thursday	Friday	Saturday
Mobility	N/A	Static Stretching	Foam Roll	Static Stretching	Foam Roll	Static Stretching	None Required
Goal	Self-Education	Establish Baseline for Push-ups, Sit-ups and 5-Mile. Record all scores	Strength and Conditioning. Record Squat score	Ranger Physical Fitness Test Focus and Speed	Strength and Conditioning. Record Deadlift score	VO2 Training and Full Body Circuit	None Required
Instructions	Recharge Mentally and Physically	None	Squat Form	POSE Running, Hamstring Activation, Intro to Turnover	Deadlift Form	POSE Running, Proper Heel Strike, Ankle Theory	Appreciate the Process
Other	Visualization – Visualize Your Future Body, You Achieving Your Goals in Body, Mind, and Spirit. Visualize Perfect Balance and Discipline (10 Minutes)	Meditate for 10 Minutes (download Headspace app for free trial)	Meditate for 10 Minutes (download Headspace app for free trial)	Meditate for 10 Minutes (download Headspace app for free trial)	Meditate for 10 Minutes (download Headspace app for free trial)	Meditate for 10 Minutes (download Headspace app for free trial)	Optional – Practice Visualization

Lesson for the Week: Be 1% BETTER

"Dominate LIFE"

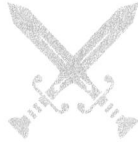

WEEK 2:
COMMAND CHANGE

Quote: *"Insanity is doing the same thing over and over, expecting a different result."* – Albert Einstein

Mission: Execute Week 2 with high intensity. By Friday, you should be broken off. Make sure you EARN IT for the weekend. This is the first week you will do a run and ruck back-to-back in the same workout. You will need running shoes and boots.

Special Instructions: Pay special attention to the purpose of each day written at the top of the program. Read each day's purpose before you start your workout. Review every workout for the week to include the instructions the day prior. Calculate your goal pace for the two-mile and five-mile events.

Mindset for the Week: This week, remind yourself that you are demanding change from your life. Every workout is about that "change." As things get hard, repeat the word "change" in your head. Tie a deep meaning to it and answer the questions: What are you changing? What are you commanding to be different? One example I use is "I am changing my behavior of settling… I will not settle."

"The Whole Man Program" WEEK 2 (High-Intensity Week)

	Sunday	Monday	Tuesday	Wednesday	Thursday	Friday	Saturday
Purpose	The Purpose of Sunday is to Reset and Refocus in a Capacity THAT WORKS FOR YOU	The Purpose of Monday Is to SWITCH IT ON	The Purpose of Tuesday Is to STACK WINS	The Purpose of Wednesday Is to GENERATE MOMENTUM	The Purpose of Thursday Is to TRY SOMETHING HARD	The Purpose of Friday Is to EARN IT FOR THE WEEKEND	The Purpose of Saturday Is to DO SOMETHING FUN OR NEW
Cardiovascular Endurance	Research Heart Rate Training Zones	3-Mile Time Trial	15 Minutes Low-impact Cardio (bike/row/walk) Heart Rate at 110-120 bpm	4-Mile Trail Run @ 80% of 3-Mile Time Trial (As a guide, add +1 min/mile to 3-Mile TT)	15 Minutes Low-impact Cardio (bike/row/walk) Heart Rate at 110-120 bpm	4 x 400m w/1:2 rest Wear athletic clothes and running shoes —then do—40-Minute Ruck Walk at 12-Mile Goal Pace Pack 35lbs Without Water Wear Athletic Clothes With Boots	Light Activity Outside or Something Fun (swimming, hiking etc..)

"The Whole Man Program" WEEK 2 (High-Intensity Week)

	Sunday	Monday	Tuesday	Wednesday	Thursday	Friday	Saturday
Strength (unless specified) • 6 Sets x 3 Reps at a weight you can complete all 6 sets with unless specified	YouTube Search CT Fletcher "The Strongest Man You Never Heard Of"	Bench Press: 5 sets x 3 Reps @75%	Back Squat: 6 sets x 3 Reps @ 75% (1 pause squat, 2 regular squat) 2:00 Rest	3 Sets Max Unbroken Pull-ups for Time	Barbell Deadlift 6 sets x 2 reps @ 75% 1RM w/2:00 Rest	None	None Required
Muscular Endurance (unless specified) • 3 Exercises per muscle group • 3-4 Sets x 15-20 Reps for Each Exercise • 30 seconds to 1 minute rest between sets • 2-3 minutes rest between exercises	Study a successful athlete of your choice	Chest and Triceps Exercises for 30 Minutes. Superset 2 Exercise for all 30 Minutes Finish with 2-3 Sets Medicine Ball Push-ups: 5 Wide, 5 Diamond, 5 Regular 30-Second Rest Between Sets, go for speed and push the limits of lactic acid buildup	20 Minutes AMRAP: 15' Rope Climb, 5 burpees, 200m Row	Back and Bicep Exercises for 30 Minutes. Superset 2 Exercise for all 30 Minutes	AMRAP 15 Minutes (KB Swing + Turkish Get-up) 10x KB Swing, 2x Turkish Get-up 15 KB Swing +2 Turkish Get-up 25 KB Swing + 2 Turkish Get-up 50 KB Swing + 2 Turkish Get-up	21-15-9 Air Squats-Push-ups-Burpees	None Required (touch on any areas of emphasis)

"The Whole Man Program" WEEK 2 (High-Intensity Week)							
	Sunday	Monday	Tuesday	Wednesday	Thursday	Friday	Saturday
Core For each Ab exercise chosen, do 3 sets to failure, rest 30 seconds between sets and 2 minutes between exercises	None	None	15 Minutes Sit-up Improvement Upper Abdominal Focus	Planks: Front, Right, Left, 3 rounds @60 seconds	15 Minutes Sit-up Improvement Lower Abdominal Focus	None	None Required
Mobility	N/A	Static Stretching	Foam Roll	Static Stretching	Foam Roll	Static Stretching	None Required
Goal	Self-Education	3-Mile Time Trial Record Time, Bench Improvement, Push-up Improvement	Strength and Conditioning	Recovery Workout	Transverse Plane Movement and Recovery Workout	2-Mile Pace Training, Ruck Conditioning, and Durability Training	None Required
Instructions	Recharge Mentally and Physically	None	Back Squat Form	Introduction To Heart Rate Training – Explanation of Target Heart Rates 120, 160, 180 bpm	Kettlebell Swing and Turkish Get-up Instruction	How to Pack and Carry a Ruck for Speed; How to Run with a Ruck	Appreciate the Process

	Sunday	Monday	Tuesday	Wednesday	Thursday	Friday	Saturday
				"The Whole Man Program" WEEK 2 (High-Intensity Week)			
Other	Visualization – Visualize Your Future Body, You Achieving Your Goals in Body, Mind, and Spirit Visualize Perfect Balance and Discipline (10 Minutes)	Meditate for 10 Minutes a day	Meditate for 10 Minutes	Meditate for 10 Minutes	Meditate for 10 Minutes	Meditate for 10 Minutes	Optional – Practice Visualization

"Dominate LIFE"

Lesson for the Week: COMMAND CHANGE

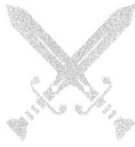

WEEK 3: BECOME DESERVING

Quote: *"The world is not a crazy enough of a place to reward a bunch of undeserving people."* – Charlie Munger

Mission: Execute Week 3 with high intensity. By Friday, you should be broken off. Make sure you EARN IT for the weekend.

Special Instructions: When studying an athlete of your choice, just learn ONE thing about them to consider the homework complete. If you want to do more, that is up to you. Keep the intensity high for the entire workout. Next week you will bring it down. Review every workout for the week to include the instructions the day prior.

Mindset for the Week: This week is about becoming DESERVING. Do not confuse deserving with entitled; you are not entitled to anything. If you apply an insane amount of work, you will get insane results. BECOME DESERVING.

	Sunday	Monday	Tuesday	Wednesday	Thursday	Friday	Saturday
"The Whole Man Program" WEEK 3 (High-Intensity Week)							
Purpose	The Purpose of Sunday is to Reset and Refocus in a Capacity THAT WORKS FOR YOU	The Purpose of Monday Is to SWITCH IT ON	The Purpose of Tuesday Is to STACK WINS	The Purpose of Wednesday Is to GENERATE MOMENTUM	The Purpose of Thursday Is to TRY SOMETHING HARD	The Purpose of Friday Is to EARN IT FOR THE WEEKEND	The Purpose of Saturday Is to DO SOMETHING FUN OR NEW
Cardiovascular Endurance	Research Heart Rate Training Zones – Calculate your Max Heart Rate. Then Calculate it at 90%, 80%, 70%, 60%, and 50%. Record in Beats Per Minute	3-Mile @ 80% of 3-Mile TT	15 Minutes Low-impact Cardio (bike/row/walk) Heart Rate at 110-120 bpm	4 x 800m at 5-Mile Goal Pace w/400m slow jog between	15 Minutes Low-impact Cardio (bike/row/walk) Heart Rate at 110-120 bpm	4-Mile Run Heart Rate at 80% max heart rate or approximately 160 bpm	Light Activity Outside or Something Fun (swimming, hiking etc.)
Strength (unless specified) • 6 Sets x 3 Reps at a weight you can complete all 6 sets with unless specified	YouTube: Mark Bell Powerlifter	Body Weight Bench Press 5 Sets @Max Reps w/2:00 Rest	Back Squat 5 Sets at 3 Reps w/2:00 Rest	4 x Max Unbroken Pull-ups (for time)	Barbell Deadlift 6 Sets x 3 Reps @ 75% 1RM w/2:00 Rest	None	None Required

"The Whole Man Program" WEEK 3 (High-Intensity Week)							
	Sunday	Monday	Tuesday	Wednesday	Thursday	Friday	Saturday
Muscular Endurance (unless specified) • **3 Exercises per muscle group** • **3-4 Sets x 15-** • **20 Reps for Each Exercise** • **30 seconds to 1 minute rest between sets** • **2-3 minutes rest between exercises**	Explore/ Research Rich Froning CrossFit Athlete	Chest and Triceps Exercises for 30 Minutes. Superset 2 Exercise for all 30 Minutes Finish with 2-3 Sets Medicine Ball Push-ups: 5 Wide, 5 Diamond, 5 Regular 30-Second Rest Between Sets, go for speed and push the limits of lactic acid buildup	14-Minute AMRAP: 7 Pull-Ups, 14 Air Squats, 7 HSPU, 14 Air Squats	Back and Bicep Exercises for 30 Minutes. Superset 2 Exercise for all 30 Minutes	For Time: 21–15–9 Dumbbell Snatch Burpees Over Dumbbell Goblet Squat (pick a weight you can complete all three rounds with – 50lbs is 'Competitive' Focus on form)	100' Handstand Walk for time OR 5 x Handstand and Hold (supported or unsupported) *If you do the handstand and hold, for each set hold for as long as comfortable then rest as long as needed – the focus is to learn how to do a proper handstand	None Required (touch on any areas of emphasis)
Core For each Ab exercise chosen, do 3 sets to failure, rest 30 seconds between sets and 2 minutes between exercises	None	None	15 Minutes Sit-up Improvement Upper Abdominal Focus	Planks: Front, Right, Left, 3 rounds @60 seconds	15 Minutes Sit-up Improvement Lower Abdominal Focus	None	None Required

177

"The Whole Man Program" WEEK 3 (High-Intensity Week)							
	Sunday	Monday	Tuesday	Wednesday	Thursday	Friday	Saturday
Mobility	None	Static Stretching	Foam Roll	Static Stretching	Foam Roll	Static Stretching	None Required
Goal	Self-Education	3-Mile Medium-Intensity Run to accumulate volume, Bench Press Strength, Push-up Improvement	Back Squat Strength, Lower Body Conditioning	VO2 Training, Pull-up Improvement, Supplementary Muscle Group Work	Recovery Cardio, Deadlift Improvement, Multiple Anatomical Plane Conditioning	4-Mile Medium-Intensity Run for Volume, Handstand Improvement, Core Conditioning	None
Instructions	Recharge Mentally and Physically	Proper Bench Press Form, Emphasis on Benching Mechanics and Direction of Force	Back Squat Form	Running Drills: Elevation drills, Running Horizontally Not Vertically	Dumbbell Snatch	How to Handstand Walk (Gymnast Method and CrossFit Method)	None
Other	Visualization – Visualize Your Future Body, You Achieving Your Goals in Body, Mind, and Spirit. Visualize Perfect Balance and Discipline (10 Minutes)	Meditate for 10 Minutes a day	Meditate for 10 Minutes	Meditate for 10 Minutes	Meditate for 10 Minutes	Meditate for 10 Minutes	Optional –Practice Visualization

"Dominate LIFE"

Lesson for the Week: BECOME DESERVING

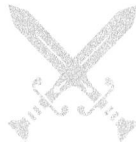

WEEK 4: ENFORCE EFFECTIVENESS

Quote: *"A man who chases two rabbits catches none."* ~ Chinese Proverb

Mission: Execute Week 4 with medium intensity. Instead of 100% effort, give 90%. However, give your max effort for the 5-mile assessment and record your time.

Special Instructions: If you have any physical agitations flaring up, treat them! Week 3 is typically the week people start to form injuries in a workout program. Become a subject matter expert in the area you are hurting the most. Treat the injury as the sport if you have one. Also, you will do legs the day before a ruck... it is intentional. Just imagine how fast you will be in the next 5-mile assessment when you have not done legs the day before.

Mindset for the Week: This week's lesson is about enforcing EFFECTIVENESS. At this point, you have the swing of the workout routine down and it is time to become more effective. Review the mind section of this book and analyze your current routine. In which areas of your life can you be more effective? How can you be more effective during your workouts and more effective with your day? Your mantra for the week is "EFFECTIVENESS."

"The Whole Man Program" WEEK 4 (Medium-Intensity Week)							
	Sunday	Monday	Tuesday	Wednesday	Thursday	Friday	Saturday
Purpose	The Purpose of Sunday is to Reset and Refocus in a Capacity THAT WORKS FOR YOU	The Purpose of Monday Is to SWITCH IT ON	The Purpose of Tuesday Is to STACK WINS	The Purpose of Wednesday Is to GENERATE MOMENTUM	The Purpose of Thursday Is to TRY SOMETHING HARD	The Purpose of Friday Is to EARN IT FOR THE WEEKEND	The Purpose of Saturday Is to DO SOMETHING FUN OR NEW
Cardiovascular Endurance	Deepen understanding of POSE Running, Arm Swing, and Hamstring Turnover Drills	30-Minute Medium-Intensity Run – Jog at the same pace for 15 min out and 15 min back Heart Rate at 70% 140 bpm	15 Minutes Low-impact Cardio (bike/row/walk) Heart Rate at 110-120 bpm	4 x 3/4-Mile (1200m) at 5-Mile Goal Pace w/400m jog as the rest	15 Minutes Low-impact Cardio (bike/row/walk) Heart Rate at 110-120 bpm	5-Mile Release Ruck March for Time (35 lbs. without water) Athletic Wear and Boots	Light Activity Outside or Something Fun (swimming, hiking etc.)
Strength (unless specified) • 6 Sets x 3 Reps at a weight you can complete all 6 sets with	YouTube/Learn One thing about Arnold Schwarzenegger	Barbell Bench Press 6 sets x 2 reps	Back Squat 6 Sets at 3 Reps w/2:00 Rest	Max Unbroken Pull-ups (record score)	Single Legged Barbell Deadlift 6 Sets x 2 Reps Each Side (Pick a weight you can control easily)	None	None Required

"The Whole Man Program" WEEK 4 (Medium-Intensity Week)							
	Sunday	Monday	Tuesday	Wednesday	Thursday	Friday	Saturday
Muscular Endurance (unless specified) • 3 Exercises per muscle group • 3-4 Sets x 15-20 Reps for Each Exercise • 30 seconds to 1 minute rest between sets • 2-3 minutes rest between exercises	Watch All or Part of *Pumping Iron* with Arnold Schwarzenegger	Chest and Triceps Exercises for 30 Minutes. Superset 2 Exercise for all 30 Minutes Finish with 2-3 Sets Medicine Ball Push-ups: 5 Wide, 5 Diamond, 5 Regular 30-Second Rest Between Sets, go for speed and push the limits of lactic acid buildup	Quadriceps Exercises for 30 Minutes Dumbbell Lunges Leg Press Hack Squat Leg Extensions Calf Raises Single Legged Calf Raises	Back and Bicep Exercises for 30 Minutes. Superset 2 Exercise for all 30 Minutes	3 Rounds 50' Overhead Lunge w/ Weight 100x Jump Rope **OR** 1:00 of Cardio Accelerator (HR 180 bpm) 50' Overhead Lunge w/Weight	10-Minute AMRAP 7 Pull-Ups 14 Air Squats 7 Toes-to-Bar 14 Push-ups (push yourself and earn it for the weekend)	None Required (touch on any areas of emphasis)
Core For each Ab exercise chosen, do 3 sets to failure, rest 30 seconds between sets and 2 minutes between exercises	None	None	15 Minutes Sit-up Improvement Upper Abdominal Focus	Planks: Front, Right, Left, 3 rounds @60 seconds	15 Minutes Sit-up Improvement Lower Abdominal Focus	None	None Required

"The Whole Man Program" WEEK 4 (Medium-Intensity Week)							
	Sunday	Monday	Tuesday	Wednesday	Thursday	Friday	Saturday
Mobility	None	Static Stretching	Foam Roll	Static Stretching	Foam Roll	Static Stretching	None Required
Goal	Study the mind of a Winner	30-Minute Medium-Intensity Run with an emphasis on sustaining pace throughout; Bench Press Strength, Push-up Improvement	Back Squat Strength, Lower Body Conditioning	VO2 Training, Pull-up Assessment, Supplementary Muscle Group Work	Recovery Cardio, Deadlift Improvement, Multiple Anatomical Plane Conditioning	5-Mile Ruck Assessment High-Intensity Training to Finish out the Week	None
Instructions	Habits of an Elite Athlete and Mindset	Pace Control	Creating a Solid Foundation for Squatting, Creating Torque in the Legs, Loading Quads,	Running Drills: Arm Swing Drills, Turnover Drills	Stiff-Legged Barbell Deadlift	Ruck Running Mechanics and Body Lean	None

"The Whole Man Program" WEEK 4 (Medium-Intensity Week)

	Sunday	Monday	Tuesday	Wednesday	Thursday	Friday	Saturday
Other	Visualization – Visualize Your Future Body, You Achieving Your Goals in Body, Mind, and Spirit. Visualize Perfect Balance and Discipline (10 Minutes)	Meditate for 10 Minutes a day	Meditate for 10 Minutes	Meditate for 10 Minutes	Meditate for 10 Minutes	Meditate for 10 Minutes	Optional –Practice Visualization

"Dominate LIFE"

Lesson for the Week: EFFECTIVENESS

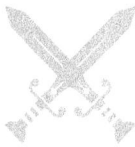

WEEK 5:
MASTER DISCIPLINE

Quote: *"To grow in life, be willing to suffer."* ~ David Goggins

Mission: Execute Week 5 with high intensity. Conduct short intervals and a forced ruck march on Friday.

Special Instructions: Rent or buy the book *Born to Run* by Christopher McDougal. Locate an area that has a pull-up bar available after your run/ruck on Friday. Focus on form for all compound lifts.

Mindset for the Week: This week's lesson is DISCIPLINE. Review the mind section of this book on discipline. Pick an area of your life in which you are going to practice growing discipline. Use this week to test your ability to control your desires. Your mantra for this week's workouts is "DISCIPLINE EQUALS FREEDOM."

"The Whole Man Program" WEEK 5 (High-Intensity Week)						
	Sunday	Monday	Tuesday	Wednesday	Thursday	Friday	Saturday
Purpose	The Purpose of Sunday is to Reset and Refocus in a Capacity THAT WORKS FOR YOU	The Purpose of Monday Is to SWITCH IT ON	The Purpose of Tuesday Is to STACK WINS	The Purpose of Wednesday Is to GENERATE MOMENTUM	The Purpose of Thursday Is to TRY SOMETHING HARD	The Purpose of Friday Is to EARN IT FOR THE WEEKEND	The Purpose of Saturday Is to DO SOMETHING FUN OR NEW
Cardiovascular Endurance	Buy and Read 1 Chapter of Born to Run by Christopher McDougall	40-Minute Medium-Intensity Run — Jog at the same pace for 20 min out and 20 min back At 80% Heart Rate (160 bpm)	15 Minutes Low-impact Cardio (bike/ row/walk) Heart Rate at 110-120 bpm	Run a 1-Mile Time Trial and rest at a 1:1 Ratio — Then do — 2 x 2 Miles at 80% Heart Rate (160 bpm)	15 Minutes Low-impact Cardio (bike/ row/walk) Heart Rate at 110-120 bpm	4 x 1/4-Mile (400m) w/200m jog in Athletic Wear and Running Shoes — Then Do — 40 Minute Conditioning Ruck March for Walk at 12-Mile Ruck Goal Pace Wear Athletic Clothes and Boots	Light Activity Outside or Something Fun (swimming, hiking etc.)

"The Whole Man Program" WEEK 5 (High-Intensity Week)

	Sunday	Monday	Tuesday	Wednesday	Thursday	Friday	Saturday
Strength (unless specified) • 6 Sets x 3 Reps at a weight you can complete all 6 sets with	YouTube: Bradley Martyn Fitness – Study Squatting Videos	Bench Press 6 sets x 2 reps @ 80% 1RM	Back Squat Do 2 reps, 1x pause, 1 regular and add weight until you work up to 2 Regular Squats at 90% 1RM	Pull-ups 4 Sets to Failure with 1:00 Rest	Clean and Press (2 Rounds): 2 Reps @ 80%, EMOM for 5:00. Rest 2:00. Repeat.	None	None Required
Muscular Endurance (unless specified) • 3 Exercises per muscle group • 3-4 Sets x 15-20 Reps for Each Exercise • 30 seconds to 1 minute rest between sets • 2-3 minutes rest between exercises	YouTube: Scott Panchik CrossFit Athlete	Chest and Triceps Exercises for 30 Minutes. Superset 2 Exercise for all 30 Minutes – Finish with 2-3 Sets Medicine Ball Push-ups: 5 Wide, 5 Diamond, 5 Regular 30 Second Rest Between Sets, go for speed and push the limits of lactic acid buildup	5 Rounds: 1:00 Goblet Squat 1:00 Wall Balls 1:00 Rest OR 1:00 Thrusters (any weight) 1:00 Cardio Accelerator (burpees, jump rope, rowing) 1:00 Rest Compete against yourself	Back and Bicep Exercises for 30 Minutes. Superset 2 Exercise for all 30 Minutes	9 Minutes AMRAP: 18 GHD Sit-ups, 12 Turkish Get-ups, 6 Overhead Squats (Easy Weight for Technique)	For Time: 50 Toes-to Bar	None Required (touch on any areas of emphasis)

"The Whole Man Program" WEEK 5 (High-Intensity Week)	Sunday	Monday	Tuesday	Wednesday	Thursday	Friday	Saturday
Core For each Ab exercise you choose do 3 sets to failure, rest 30 seconds between sets and 2 minutes between exercises	None	None	15 Minutes Sit-up Improvement Upper Abdominal Focus	Planks: Front, Right, Left, 3 rounds @60 seconds	15 Minutes Sit-up Improvement Lower Abdominal Focus	None	None Required
Mobility	None	Static Stretching	Foam Roll	Static Stretching	Foam Roll	Static Stretching	None Required
Goal	Study Winners	40-Minute Medium-Intensity Run with an emphasis on sustaining pace throughout; Bench Press Strength, Push-up Improvement	Back Squat Strength, Lower Body Conditioning	VO2 Training, Pull-up Improvement, Supplementary Muscle Group Work	Compound Movements, Multiple Anatomical Plan Training	Pace Training, Ruck Conditioning, Training for Durability	None

"The Whole Man Program" WEEK 5 (High-Intensity Week)

	Sunday	Monday	Tuesday	Wednesday	Thursday	Friday	Saturday
Instructions	The Tarahumara	Pace Control	Pause Squats	Concentric vs Eccentric Muscle Contraction	Overhead Squats, Clean and Press	Nutrition – Power of General Rules Beating Any Diet	None
Other	Visualization – Visualize Your Future Body, You Achieving Your Goals in Body, Mind, and Spirit. Visualize Perfect Balance and Discipline (10 Minutes)	Meditate for 10 Minutes a day	Meditate for 10 Minutes	Meditate for 10 Minutes	Meditate for 10 Minutes	Meditate for 10 Minutes	Optional –Practice Visualization

"Dominate LIFE"

Lesson for the Week: DISCIPLINE EQUALS FREEDOM

189

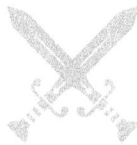

WEEK 6: CREATE SPECIFICITY

Quote: *"Your focus determines your reality."* ~ George Lucas

Mission: Execute Week 6 with high intensity. Give your max effort for the 5-mile assessment and record your time.

Special Instructions: Friday's workout will be tough. When you finish, praise yourself for your hard work. Put emphasis on meditation and visualization this week. Create an image of your future self.

Mindset for the Week: This week's lesson is SPECIFICITY. Create a character in your mind of who you are trying to become — a visual depiction of you at your greatest self. Once complete, give the image of your future self a name. As an example, Charlie Jabaley is a music manager who changed career paths to becoming a Nike athlete. When he decided to change directions in life, he changed the nickname he had for himself. He went from "CEO Charlie" to "Charlie Rocket" to manifest his desires. What does your future self look like? How do they act? What are their physical capabilities? Your mantra for the week is "SPECIFICITY" – every time you think it or say it, imagine being the character you have created.

"The Whole Man Program" WEEK 6 (High-Intensity Week)							
	Sunday	Monday	Tuesday	Wednesday	Thursday	Friday	Saturday
Purpose	The Purpose of Sunday is to Reset and Refocus in a Capacity THAT WORKS FOR YOU	The Purpose of Monday Is to SWITCH IT ON	The Purpose of Tuesday Is to STACK WINS	The Purpose of Wednesday Is to GENERATE MOMENTUM	The Purpose of Thursday Is to TRY SOMETHING HARD	The Purpose of Friday Is to EARN IT FOR THE WEEKEND	The Purpose of Saturday Is to DO SOMETHING FUN OR NEW
Cardiovascular Endurance	Read 1 Chapter of *Born to Run* by Christopher McDougall	5-Mile Time Trial. Record Score	15 Minutes Low-impact Cardio (bike/row/walk) Heart Rate at 110-120 bpm	4 x 3/4 Mile (1200m) at 5-Mile Goal Pace w/3:00 Rest	15 Minutes Low-impact Cardio (bike/row/walk) Heart Rate at 110-120 bpm	60-Minute Ruck Run (30 minutes out and 30 minutes back), Jog for 3:00 then Walk for 3:00. Repeat for Entire Workout (Wear Athletic Clothes and Boots)	Light Activity Outside or Something Fun (swimming, hiking etc.)
Strength (unless specified) • 6 Sets x 3 Reps at a weight you can complete all 6 sets with	YouTube: Mark Bell Bench Press	Bench Press 6 sets x 2 reps add 5lbs from last week	Front Squat 5 Sets x 3 Reps	Max Pull-ups in 5 Minutes	Military Press (DB or BB), 5 Sets x 5 Reps	None	None Required

"The Whole Man Program" WEEK 6 (High-Intensity Week)

	Sunday	Monday	Tuesday	Wednesday	Thursday	Friday	Saturday
Muscular Endurance (unless specified) 3 Exercises per muscle group 3-4 Sets x 15-20 Reps for Each Exercise 30 seconds to 1 minute rest between sets 2-3 minutes rest between exercises	YouTube: Michael Jordan's "The Flu Game"	Chest and Triceps Exercises for 30 Minutes. Superset 2 Exercise for all 30 Minutes-Finish with 2-3 Sets Medicine Ball Push-ups: 5 Wide, 5 Diamond, 5 Regular 30 Second Rest Between Sets, go for speed and push the limits of lactic acid buildup	5 Rounds: 12 x Deadlifts 24 x Step Ups 12 x Second Hold on Peg Board or Pull-up Bar	Back and Bicep Exercises for 30 Minutes. Superset 2 Exercise for all 30 Minutes	Rounds: x Barbell Deadlifts 5 x Hang Power Cleans 5 x Front Squats 5 x Push Press Rest 2:00	For Time: 12-9-6-3 Burpee, Toes To Bar, Push-ups	None Required (touch on any areas of emphasis)
Core For each Ab exercise you choose do 3 sets to failure, rest 30 seconds between sets and 2 minutes between exercises	None	None	15 Minutes Sit-up Improvement Upper Abdominal Focus	Planks: Front, Right, Left, 3 rounds @60 seconds	15 Minutes Sit-up Improvement Lower Abdominal Focus	None	None Required

194

"The Whole Man Program" WEEK 6 (High-Intensity Week)							
	Sunday	Monday	Tuesday	Wednesday	Thursday	Friday	Saturday
Mobility	None	Static Stretching	Foam Roll	Static Stretching	Foam Roll	Static Stretching	None Required
Goal	Study Winners	40-Minute Medium-Intensity Run with an emphasis on sustaining pace throughout; Bench Press Strength, Push-up Improvement	Front Squat Strength, Lower Body Conditioning	VO2 Training, Pull-up Improvement, Supplementary Muscle Group Work	Compound Movements	Pace Training, Ruck Conditioning, Training for Durability	None
Instructions	Introduction to the book *Relentless* Michael Jordan as a cleaner	Pace Control	Front Squat	Introduction to Fitness Programming and the B.O.D.Y. Concept	Hang Power Cleans, Push Press	"Feel Good Runs" – How Negative Reinforcement Creates Negative Associations to Cardio	None

	Sunday	Monday	Tuesday	Wednesday	Thursday	Friday	Saturday
				"The Whole Man Program" WEEK 6 (High-Intensity Week)			
Other	Visualization – Visualize Your Future Body, You Achieving Your Goals in Body, Mind, and Spirit. Visualize Perfect Balance and Discipline (10 Minutes)	Meditate for 10 Minutes a day	Meditate for 10 Minutes	Meditate for 10 Minutes	Meditate for 10 Minutes	Meditate for 10 Minutes	Optional –Practice Visualization

Lesson for the Week: SPECIFICITY

"Dominate LIFE"

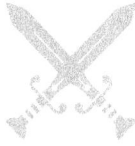

WEEK 7: HABITS MAKE US

Quote: *"The chains of habit are too light to be felt until they are too heavy to be broken."* ~ Warren Buffett

Mission: Execute Week 7 with medium intensity. Give Monday and Wednesday your attention this week and focus on "time under tension." Review next week's 1RM schedule.

Special Instructions: On Sunday, research the Habit Loop by Charles Duhigg and share it with somebody to reinforce your understanding. Apply the Tarahumara mindset from the book *Born to Run*. Add it to your runs and "think easy, light and smooth" – as the author states. Research "time under tension" and apply it to Monday's and Wednesday's workouts.

Mindset for the Week: This week's lesson is about HABITS. We are what we repeatedly do. Observe your current habits and rituals this week. As a challenge, try to discover a habit you did not know you had. As you work out this week, your mantra is "Habits Make Us." Feel proud that you are controlling your habits now, that you are creating them and not becoming a victim of them. Habits are yours to command.

THE WHOLE MAN PROJECT

"The Whole Man Program" WEEK 7 (Medium-Intensity Week)							
	Sunday	Monday	Tuesday	Wednesday	Thursday	Friday	Saturday
Purpose	The Purpose of Sunday is to Reset and Refocus in a Capacity THAT WORKS FOR YOU	The Purpose of Monday Is to SWITCH IT ON	The Purpose of Tuesday Is to STACK WINS	The Purpose of Wednesday Is to GENERATE MOMENTUM	The Purpose of Thursday Is to TRY SOMETHING HARD	The Purpose of Friday Is to EARN IT FOR THE WEEKEND	The Purpose of Saturday Is to DO SOMETHING FUN OR NEW
Cardiovascular Endurance	Continue to Read *Born to Run* by Christopher McDougall	Run 3 Miles at 85% of Max HR (165-170 bpm)	15 Minutes Low-impact Cardio (bike/row/walk) Heart Rate at 110-120 bpm	4 x 3/4Mile (1200m) at 5-Mile Goal Pace w/3:00 Rest	15 Minutes Low-impact Cardio (bike/row/walk) Heart Rate at 110-120 bpm	4 x 1/4-Mile (400m) at 2-Mile Goal Pace w/400m jog between (wear athletic clothes and running shoes) — Then Do — 30Min Ruck, 15 Min Out/15 Min Back w/35Lbs without water (wear athletic clothes and boots)	Light Activity Outside or Something Fun (swimming, hiking etc.)

"The Whole Man Program" WEEK 7 (Medium-Intensity Week)

	Sunday	Monday	Tuesday	Wednesday	Thursday	Friday	Saturday
Strength (unless specified) • **6 Sets x 3 Reps at a weight you can complete all 6 sets with**	Download 1 interesting audio on either iTunes or Soundcloud by Barbell Shrugged	Bench Press 5 Sets x 3 Reps @ 80% of 1RM	Back Squat 5 Sets x 3 Reps (Time Under Tension 4-2-2-1)	4 Sets Max Pull-ups w/1:00 Rest (kipping is OK once you are near failure)	Standing Dumbbell or Barbell Military Press (pick the opposite of last week) 5 Sets x 5 Reps	None	None Required
Muscular Endurance (unless specified) • **3 Exercises per muscle group** • **3-4 Sets x 15-20 Reps for Each Exercise** • **30 seconds to 1 minute rest between sets** • **2-3 minutes rest between exercises**	Discover and Research Athlete of Choice	Chest and Triceps Exercises for 30 Minutes. Superset 2 Exercise for all 30 Minutes – Finish with 2-3 Sets Medicine Ball Push-ups: 5 Wide, 5 Diamond, 5 Regular 30 Second Rest Between Sets, go for speed and push the limits of lactic acid buildup	18 Min AMRAP 10 Front Squat 20 Push-ups 10 KB Swing 20 Single Arm Overhead Walk w/KB 10 Pull-ups 20 Lunges 10 Stairs 20 V-ups 10 Wall Balls 20 (4 count) Combat Rope 10 Sit-ups 20 Step-ups or Box Jumps	Back and Bicep Exercises for 30 Minutes. Superset 2 Exercise for all 30 Minutes	For Time: 30 Deadlifts @ BW, 30 Pull-ups, 30 Calorie Bike or Row	10-Minute AMRAP 15 Push-ups 20 Air Squats 25 V-ups 30 Lunges	None Required (touch on any areas of emphasis)

	Sunday	Monday	Tuesday	Wednesday	Thursday	Friday	Saturday
"The Whole Man Program" WEEK 7 (Medium-Intensity Week)							
Core For each Ab exercise you choose do 3 sets to failure, rest 30 seconds between sets and 2 minutes between exercises	None	None	15 Minutes Sit-up Improvement Upper Abdominal Focus	Planks: Front, Right, Left, 3 rounds @60 seconds	15 Minutes Sit-up Improvement Lower Abdominal Focus	None	None Required
Mobility	None	Static Stretching	Foam Roll	Static Stretching	Foam Roll	Static Stretching	None Required
Goal	Inspire Yourself	Heart Rate Run, Bench Press Improvement	Back Squat Strength, Lower Body and core Conditioning	VO2 Training, Pull-up Improvement, Supplementary Muscle Group Work	Shoulder Improvement, Core Work, Deadlift Improvement	Pace Training, Ruck Conditioning, Training for Durability	None
Instructions	The Habit Loop – Cue, Routine Reward	Emphasis on "Feel Good Runs" and the Tarahumara mindset – Think Easy, Light and Smooth	Time Under Tension	Time Under Tension	Hang Power Cleans, Push Press	How to Break the Habit Loop (Charles Duhigg)	None

"The Whole Man Program" WEEK 7 (Medium-Intensity Week)

	Sunday	Monday	Tuesday	Wednesday	Thursday	Friday	Saturday
Other	Visualization – Visualize Your Future Body, You Achieving Your Goals in Body, Mind, and Spirit. Visualize Perfect Balance and Discipline (10 Minutes)	Meditate for 10 Minutes a day	Meditate for 10 Minutes	Meditate for 10 Minutes	Meditate for 10 Minutes	Meditate for 10 Minutes	Optional –Practice Visualization

"Dominate LIFE"

Lesson for the Week: HABITS MAKE US

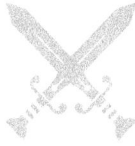

WEEK 8: TEST DAYS

Quote: *"Love the Test Days."* ~ Andy Frisella

Mission: Execute Week 8 with high intensity. Give max effort for all lifts and analyze your results.

Special Instructions: Record all of your 1RM and compare them to the start of the program. Analyze what you think worked well and what did not so that you can improve from the lessons learned. The focus for the rest of the program is the Ranger Physical Fitness Test (RPFT) and 12-mile ruck. This is the last time you will do a 1RM in this program. Your next opportunity will be on your own after its completion.

Mindset for the Week: This week's lesson is about "TEST DAYS." Andy Frisella from the 1st Phorm Supplements and The MFCEO Project calls the days you do not feel like doing something "Test Days." Testing yourself during your weakest moment is the measure of who you are and what you are made of. At this point of the program, you have stacked up 50 days of being 1% better. Congratulations, you are more than 50% better than when you started, in both body and mind. Time to test yourself; every day this week, execute your workouts with the mental mantra "TEST DAY."

"The Whole Man Program" WEEK 8 (High-Intensity Week)

	Sunday	Monday	Tuesday	Wednesday	Thursday	Friday	Saturday
Purpose	The Purpose of Sunday is to Reset and Refocus in a Capacity THAT WORKS FOR YOU	The Purpose of Monday Is to SWITCH IT ON	The Purpose of Tuesday Is to STACK WINS	The Purpose of Wednesday Is to GENERATE MOMENTUM	The Purpose of Thursday Is to TRY SOMETHING HARD	The Purpose of Friday Is to EARN IT FOR THE WEEKEND	The Purpose of Saturday Is to DO SOMETHING FUN OR NEW
Cardiovascular Endurance	Continue to Read *Born to Run* by Christopher McDougall	Run 6 Miles at 80% of 5-Mile Time Trial	15 Minutes Low-impact Cardio (bike/row/walk) Heart Rate at 110–120 bpm	4 x 3/4Mile (1200m) at 5-Mile Goal Pace w/3:00 Rest	15 Minutes Low-impact Cardio (bike/row/walk) Heart Rate at 110–120 bpm	8 x 1/4-Mile w/1:1 Rest; Run at 2-Mile Goal Pace — Then Do — 40-Min Ruck Run 20 Min Out/20 at 3:00 Jog then 3:00 Walk – Do not go slower than 15-minute-mile pace during the walk – Use w/35 lbs. without water	Light Activity Outside or Something NEW (swimming, hiking etc.)

"The Whole Man Program" WEEK 8 (High-Intensity Week)

	Sunday	Monday	Tuesday	Wednesday	Thursday	Friday	Saturday
Strength (unless specified) • **6 Sets x 3 Reps at a weight you can complete all 6 sets with**	Download and Listen to 1 interesting audio on either iTunes or Soundcloud by *The Model Health Show* – Shawn Stevenson	1RM Bench Press (Record)	1RM Back Squat (Record)	Max Pull-up (Record)	Deadlift 1RM (Record)	None	None Required
Muscular Endurance (unless specified) • **3 Exercises per muscle group** • **3-4 Sets x 15-20 Reps for Each Exercise** • **30 seconds to 1 minute rest between sets** • **2-3 minutes rest between exercises**	Discover and Research Athlete of Choice	Chest and Triceps Exercises for 30 Minutes. Superset 2 Exercise for all 30 Minutes – Finish with 2-3 Sets Medicine Ball Push-ups: 5 Wide, 5 Diamond, 5 Regular 30 Second Rest Between Sets, go for speed and push the limits of lactic acid buildup	3 Rounds For Time: 10 x Overhead Squat 25' Sled Push and/or Pull w/180 lbs. 50' Overhead Plate Walk	Back and Bicep Exercises for 30 Minutes. Superset 2 Exercise for all 30 Minutes	For Time: 10-9-8-7-6-5-4-3-2-1 Lunges + KB Swing	For Time: 25 Toes-To-Bar	None Required (touch on any areas of emphasis)

"The Whole Man Program" WEEK 8 (High-Intensity Week)

	Sunday	Monday	Tuesday	Wednesday	Thursday	Friday	Saturday
Core For each Ab exercise you choose do 3 sets to failure, rest 30 seconds between sets and 2 minutes between exercises	None	None	15 Minutes Sit-up Improvement Upper Abdominal Focus	Planks: Front, Right, Left, 3 rounds @60 seconds	15 Minutes Sit-up Improvement Lower Abdominal Focus	None	None Required
Mobility	None	Static Stretching	Foam Roll	Static Stretching	Foam Roll	Static Stretching	None Required
Goal	Self-Education	1 Rep Max Assessment	1 Rep Max Assessment, Light Circuit	Max Pull-up Assessment	1 Rep Max Assessment, Light Circuit	Pace Training, Ruck Conditioning, Training for Durability	None
Instructions	None	Analysis of Max Assessment to Week 1	Analysis of Max Assessment to Week 1	Analysis of Max Assessment to Week 1	Analysis of Max Assessment to Week 1	Goal Paces for 3:00/3:00 Training	None

"The Whole Man Program" WEEK 8 (High-Intensity Week)						
	Sunday	Monday	Tuesday	Wednesday	Thursday	Friday	Saturday
Other	Visualization – Visualize Your Future Body, You Achieving Your Goals in Body, Mind, and Spirit. Visualize Perfect Balance and Discipline (10 Minutes)	Meditate for 10 Minutes a day	Meditate for 10 Minutes	Meditate for 10 Minutes	Meditate for 10 Minutes	Meditate for 10 Minutes	Optional –Practice Visualization

"Dominate LIFE"

Lesson for the Week: TEST DAYS

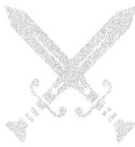

WEEK 9:
ALL THINGS ARE EASY

Quote: *"All things are easy"* ~ Charlie Jabaley

Mission: Execute Week 9 with high intensity. Give max effort for all lifts and analyze your results.

Special Instructions: Review the nutrition section of this book. Create new eating rules. Read one passage from the discipline section of this program. Identify one thing in your life that once took a lot of discipline but has become easy.

Mindset for the Week: This week's lesson is "IT IS EASY." Charlie Jabaley is a music manager turned Nike athlete. Read and digest his thoughts on things that are hard every day this week. Enforce the belief "it is EASY" into your workouts.

I go into everything with the thought process of "it is easy," because, at one time in our life, walking was very, very hard. But if we look back on it, it was a process. It was hard, and then we kind of did it, and did it, and did it... and then all of a sudden, it is easy. So, if we know that is how everything works—whether it is multiplication, division, walking, tying our shoe—if all these things were at one point hard and ended up being easy—and we know that is how it works every single time—we're always going to end up saying "it is easy." So why not just say that for everything?

"The Whole Man Program" WEEK 9 (High-Intensity Week)

	Sunday	Monday	Tuesday	Wednesday	Thursday	Friday	Saturday
Purpose	The Purpose of Sunday is to Reset and Refocus in a Capacity THAT WORKS FOR YOU	The Purpose of Monday Is to SWITCH IT ON	The Purpose of Tuesday Is to STACK WINS	The Purpose of Wednesday Is to GENERATE MOMENTUM	The Purpose of Thursday Is to TRY SOMETHING HARD	The Purpose of Friday Is to EARN IT FOR THE WEEKEND	The Purpose of Saturday Is to DO SOMETHING FUN OR NEW
Cardiovascular Endurance	Continue to Read *Born to Run* by Christopher McDougall	5-Mile at 90% of 5-Mile Time Trial	15 Minutes Low-impact Cardio (bike/row/walk) Heart Rate at 110-120 bpm	4x 1/2Mile (800m) at 5-Mile Goal Pace w/2:00 Rest Between Each	15 Minutes Low-impact Cardio (bike/row/walk) Heart Rate at 110-120 bpm	6 x 1/4-Mile (400m) w/200m jog at 90% Max Heart Rate (180 bpm) wear athletic clothes and running shoes —Then Do— 40-Min Ruck 20-Min Out/20 min back- Use w/35Lbs without water (athletic clothes and boots)	Light Activity Outside or Something NEW (swimming, hiking, etc.)

"The Whole Man Program" WEEK 9 (High-Intensity Week)

	Sunday	Monday	Tuesday	Wednesday	Thursday	Friday	Saturday
Strength (unless specified) • **6 Sets x 3 Reps at a weight you can complete all 6 sets with**	Download and Listen to 1 interesting audio on either iTunes or Soundcloud by Fitness Podcast of Choice	Dumbbell Bench Press: 5 sets x 3 Reps @75%	Back Squat: 6 sets x 3 Reps @ 75% 1RM (1 pause squat, 2 regular squat) 2:00 Rest	Pull-ups 5 Unbroken Sets to Failure w/30 seconds of rest	Military Press (DB or BB), 5 Sets x 5 Reps	None	None Required
Muscular Endurance (unless specified) • **3 Exercises per muscle group** • **3-4 Sets x 15-20 Reps for Each Exercise** • **30 seconds to 1 minute rest between sets** • **2-3 minutes rest between exercises**	Discover and Research Athlete of Choice (use any platform available, Instagram, Snapchat, or the internet). Learn Something new about weightlifting	Chest and Triceps Exercises for 30 Minutes. Do 3 Chest Exercises then 3 Triceps Exercise for 30 Minutes – Finish with 2-3 Sets Medicine Ball Push-ups: 10 Wide, 10 Diamond, 10 Regular 30 Second Rest Between Sets, go for speed and push the limits of lactic acid buildup	4 Rounds For Time 25' KB Lunges 20 Toes to Bar or Leg Raises, 15 Dumbbell Press, 10 Burpees	Back and Bicep Exercises for 30 Minutes. Do 3 Back Exercises then do 3 bicep Exercises for 30 Minutes	Every Minute On the Minute: 6 x Dumbbell Squat Clean + 1 Rope Climb (20')	30-20-10 Toes to Bar Push-ups 7:00 Time Cap	None Required (touch on any areas of emphasis)

"The Whole Man Program" WEEK 9 (High-Intensity Week)							
	Sunday	Monday	Tuesday	Wednesday	Thursday	Friday	Saturday
Core For each Ab exercise you choose do 3 sets to failure, rest 30 seconds between sets and 2 minutes between exercises	None	None	15 Minutes Sit-up Improvement Upper Abdominal Focus	Planks: Front, Right, Left, 3 rounds @60 seconds	15 Minutes Sit-up Improvement Lower Abdominal Focus	None	None Required
Mobility	None	Static Stretching	Foam Roll	Static Stretching	Foam Roll	Static Stretching	None Required
Goal	Self-Education	Bench Press Improvement and Progressive Overload	Back Squat Improvement, High-Intensity Circuit	Pull-up Improvement, VO2 Training	Shoulder Improvement, Rope Climb, High-Intensity Circuit	Pace Training, Ruck Conditioning, Training for Durability	None
Instructions	Individual Discipline in Self-Study	How discipline and decisions have "fuel tanks"	Kettlebell Lunges	Running Mechanics at Longer Distances, Checking in with the Body During a Run	Dumbbell Squat Clean, Rope Climb Technique	Nutrition and Rules	None

213

"The Whole Man Program" WEEK 9 (High-Intensity Week)						
	Sunday	Monday	Tuesday	Wednesday	Thursday	Friday	Saturday
Other	Visualization – Visualize Your Future Body, You Achieving Your Goals in Body, Mind, and Spirit. Visualize Perfect Balance and Discipline (10 Minutes)	Meditate for 10 Minutes a day	Meditate for 10 Minutes	Meditate for 10 Minutes	Meditate for 10 Minutes	Meditate for 10 Minutes	Optional –Practice Visualization

"Dominate LIFE"

Lesson for the Week: IT'S EASY

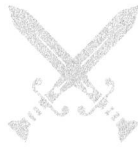

WEEK 10:
SELF-TRUST

Quote: *"Confidence is built by creating self-trust"* ~ Ed Mylett

Mission: Execute Week 12 with medium intensity. Give max effort for all lifts and analyze your results.

Special Instructions: This week begins our taper; you will do the Army Ranger Physical Fitness Test in Week 11, and the final ruck in Week 12. The most difficult workout for the week will be Friday. You will do short intervals and a ruck run.

Mindset for the Week: This week's lesson is about "SELF-TRUST." Ed Mylett is the Agency Chairman of World Financial Group and a renowned motivational speaker. He states that in order to generate confidence, we have to live up to the private promises we make to ourselves. Living up to our word creates SELF-TRUST and turns into confidence. This week, every work-out is about living up to your word and creating SELF-TRUST.

"The Whole Man Program" WEEK 10 (Medium-Intensity Week)							
	Sunday	Monday	Tuesday	Wednesday	Thursday	Friday	Saturday
Purpose	The Purpose of Sunday is to Reset and Refocus in a Capacity THAT WORKS FOR YOU	The Purpose of Monday Is to SWITCH IT ON	The Purpose of Tuesday Is to STACK WINS	The Purpose of Wednesday Is to GENERATE MOMENTUM	The Purpose of Thursday Is to TRY SOMETHING HARD	The Purpose of Friday Is to EARN IT FOR THE WEEKEND	The Purpose of Saturday Is to DO SOMETHING FUN OR NEW
Cardiovascular Endurance	Continue to Read *Born to Run* by Christopher McDougall	30-Minute Recovery Run 15min out/15 min back (HR ~160 bpm)	15 Minutes Low-impact Cardio (bike/row/walk) Heart Rate at 110-120 bpm	4x1/4Mile (400m) @ 70% Max Heart Rate w/200m Jog	15 Minutes Low-impact Cardio (bike/row/walk) Heart Rate at 110-120 bpm	12 x 200m w/2:00 Rest wear Athletic Clothes and Running Shoes —Then Do— 40-Min Ruck Run 20-Min Out/20 min back with 3:00 Jog and 3:00 Walk – w/40Lbs without water (field uniform and boots)	Light Activity Outside or Something NEW (swimming, hiking etc.)

	Sunday	Monday	Tuesday	Wednesday	Thursday	Friday	Saturday
Strength (unless specified) • **6 Sets x 3 Reps at a weight you can complete all 6 sets with**	Download and Listen to 1 interesting audio on either iTunes or SoundCloud by Fitness Podcast of Choice	Bench Press 6 Sets x 2 Reps (add 5lbs from last week)	Back Squat 5 Sets x 5 Reps	Max Pull-ups in 5 Minutes (kipping allowed once you reach failure)	Military Press (DB or BB), 5 Sets x 5 Reps	None	None Required
Muscular Endurance (unless specified) • **3 Exercises per muscle group** • **3-4 Sets x 15-20 Reps for Each Exercise** • **30 seconds to 1 minute rest between sets** • **2-3 minutes rest between exercises**	Discover and Research Athlete of Choice (use any platform available, Instagram, Snapchat, or the internet) Learn Something new about weightlifting	Chest and Triceps Exercises for 30 Minutes. Do 3 Chest Exercises then 3 Triceps Exercise for 30 Minutes- Finish with 2-3 Sets Medicine Ball Push-ups: 10 Wide, 10 Diamond, 10 Regular 30 Second Rest Between Sets, go for speed and push the limits of lactic acid buildup	5 Rounds: 12 Deadlifts 24 Step Ups or Box Jumps 12 Second Hold (Peg Board or Pull-up Bar)	Back and Bicep Exercises for 30 Minutes. Do 3 Back Exercises then do 3 bicep Exercises for 30 Minutes	Rounds: Deadlifts 5 Hang Power Cleans 5 Front Squats 5 Push Press Rest 2:00	5 Rounds for Time: 5 Pull-ups 10 Push-ups 15 Air Squats	None Required (touch on any areas of emphasis)

"The Whole Man Program" WEEK 10 (Medium-Intensity Week)

"The Whole Man Program" WEEK 10 (Medium-Intensity Week)

	Sunday	Monday	Tuesday	Wednesday	Thursday	Friday	Saturday
Core For each Ab exercise you choose do 3 sets to failure, rest 30 seconds between sets and 2 minutes between exercises	None	None	15 Minutes Sit-up Improvement Upper Abdominal Focus	Planks: Front, Right, Left, 3 rounds @60 seconds	15 Minutes Sit-up Improvement Lower Abdominal Focus	None	None Required
Mobility	None	Static Stretching	Foam Roll	Static Stretching	Foam Roll	Static Stretching	None Required
Goal	Self-Education	Taper Week	Taper Week	Taper Week	Taper Week	High-Intensity Workout For the Week, Pace Training, Ruck Conditioning, Training for Durability	None
Instructions	Individual Discipline in Self-Study	Treat Days vs Cheat Days	Push-up and Sit-up Strategy Discussion for APFT	Lung Capacity and How to Regain Breath During Runs, Front Loading Oxygen	Hang Power Cleans, Front Squats	How to Transition Mentally and Physically Between Multiple Endurance Events	None

"The Whole Man Program" WEEK 10 (Medium-Intensity Week)

	Sunday	Monday	Tuesday	Wednesday	Thursday	Friday	Saturday
Other	Visualization – Visualize Your Future Body, You Achieving Your Goals in Body, Mind, and Spirit. Visualize Perfect Balance and Discipline (10 Minutes)	Meditate for 10 Minutes a day	Meditate for 10 Minutes	Meditate for 10 Minutes	Meditate for 10 Minutes	Meditate for 10 Minutes	Optional –Practice Visualization

"Dominate LIFE"

Lesson for the Week: SELF-TRUST

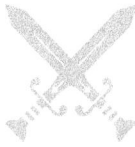

WEEK 11: EMBRACE FEAR

Quote: *"The best things in life are on the other side of fear."* ~ Will Smith

Mission: Execute Week 11 with medium intensity on Monday through Thursday. Conduct the Ranger Physical Fitness Test (RPFT) on Friday.

Special Instructions: Give your max effort on Friday and record your results. Compare your scores against the beginning of the program. Review all of the RPFT standards, review "Treat Days" vs. "Cheat Days" and plan a treat for the end of the program.

Mindset for the Week: This week's lesson is about "FEAR." Giving something your all is intimidating. Most people cannot do it and leave a little bit of commitment in reserve so they have something to blame in case they do not meet their

221

goal. You will hear people saying, "Well, it's a good thing I didn't try" when they fail at something. The idea that they did not try is a copout. It gives them a "justifiable" excuse for failing and protects their ego. This week is about stepping into fear. Accept you are going to go all in, regardless of the outcome. During your workouts, recite "EMBRACE FEAR" over and over as a method of conquering it.

"The Whole Man Program" WEEK 11 (Medium-Intensity and RPFT)							
	Sunday	Monday	Tuesday	Wednesday	Thursday	Friday	Saturday
Purpose	The Purpose of Sunday is to Reset and Refocus in a Capacity THAT WORKS FOR YOU	The Purpose of Monday Is to SWITCH IT ON	The Purpose of Tuesday Is to STACK WINS	The Purpose of Wednesday Is to GENERATE MOMENTUM	The Purpose of Thursday Is to TRY SOMETHING HARD	The Purpose of Friday Is to EARN IT FOR THE WEEKEND	The Purpose of Saturday Is to DO SOMETHING FUN OR NEW
Cardiovascular Endurance	Continue to Read *Born to Run* by Christopher McDougall	30-Minute Recovery Run 15min out/15 min back (HR ~160 bpm)	15 Minutes Low-impact Cardio (bike/row/walk) Heart Rate at 110-120 bpm	30-Minute Run at 80% max heart rate (160 bpm)	15 Minutes Low-impact Cardio (bike/row/walk) Heart Rate at 110-120 bpm	Ranger Physical Fitness Test 2:00 Push-ups Max Effort	Light Activity Outside or Something NEW (swimming, hiking etc.)
Strength (unless specified) • 6 Sets x 3 Reps at a weight you can complete all 6 sets with	Download and Listen to 1 interesting audio on either iTunes or Soundcloud by Fitness Podcast of Choice	Bench Press 6 Sets x 2 Reps (add 5lbs from last week)	Overhead Squats 5 Sets x 5 Reps @ Difficult Weight (Time Under Tension (Time Under Tension 4-2-2-1)	Barbell Row 5 Sets x 5 Reps @ Difficult Weight	Single Legged Deadlift: 5 sets x 5 reps With Light Weight	2:00 Sit-ups Max Effort 5-Mile Timed Run Max Effort Max Pull-ups Unbroken (Record)	None Required

"The Whole Man Program" WEEK 11 (Medium-Intensity and RPFT)

	Sunday	Monday	Tuesday	Wednesday	Thursday	Friday	Saturday
Muscular Endurance (unless specified) • 3 Exercises per muscle group • 3-4 Sets x 15-20 Reps for Each Exercise • 30 seconds to 1 minute rest between sets • 2-3 minutes rest between exercises	Discover and Research Athlete of Choice (use any platform available, Instagram, Snapchat, or the internet) Learn something new about weightlifting	Chest and Triceps Exercises for 20 Minutes. Do 3 Chest Exercises then 3 Triceps Exercises (Light Weight for Entire Workout – Stimulate the Muscle Groups But do not Fatigue Them)	For Time: 100 Calorie Row 75 Thrusters 50 Pull-Ups 75 Wall Ball Shots or Similar 100 Calorie Row	Back and Bicep Exercises for 20 Minutes. Do 2 Back Exercises then do 2 bicep Exercises for 30 Minutes	6 Rounds: 1K Bike or Row 25 KB Swings Easy Intensity	Ranger Physical Fitness Test 2:00 Push-ups Max Effort 2:00 Sit-ups Max Effort 5-Mile Timed Run Max Effort Max Pull-ups Unbroken (Record)	None Required (touch on any areas of emphasis)
Core For each Ab exercise you choose do 3 sets to failure, rest 30 seconds between sets and 2 minutes between exercises	None	Planks: Front, Right, Left, 3 rounds @60 seconds	15 Minutes Sit-up Improvement Upper Abdominal Focus	None	None		None Required

"The Whole Man Program" WEEK 11 (Medium-Intensity and RPFT)

	Sunday	Monday	Tuesday	Wednesday	Thursday	Friday	Saturday
Mobility	None	Static Stretching	Foam Roll	Static Stretching	Foam Roll	Static Stretching	None Required
Goal	Self-Education	Taper	Taper	Taper	Taper	RPFT Max Effort	None
Instructions	Individual Discipline in Self-Study	Treat Days vs Cheat Days	RPFT Standards Overview	Lung Capacity and How to Regain Breath During Runs, Front Loading Oxygen	Single Legged Deadlift	RPFT Standards	None
Other	Visualization – Visualize Your Future Body, You Achieving Your Goals in Body, Mind, and Spirit. Visualize Perfect Balance and Discipline (10 Minutes)	Meditate for 10 Minutes a day	Meditate for 10 Minutes	Meditate for 10 Minutes	Meditate for 10 Minutes	Meditate for 10 Minutes	Optional –Practice Visualization

"Dominate LIFE"

Lesson for the Week: EMBRACE FEAR

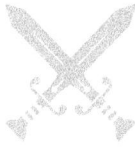

WEEK 12: SUCCESS

Quote: *"Success is an inside job."* ~ James Allen

Mission: Execute Week 12 with medium intensity on Monday and Tuesday. Then give 100% effort on the 12-mile ruck.

Special Instructions: Prepare yourself for the 12-mile ruck. Break down how you will tackle each mile and what your nutrition plan will be. Research foot care. Research how ultra-marathon runners tend to their feet.

Mindset for the Week: This week's lesson is about "SUCCESS." Accomplishing our goals comes down to mindset. Are we willing to put in the work? Are we willing to give it our all? Are we willing to think we are capable and not make excuses in the pursuit? Every day this week, take ownership of your outcome and remind yourself you are responsible for what happens. Repeat the mantra "SUCCESS" in your head as things get difficult. Rehearse it daily. Take ownership. Success is an inside job.

	Sunday	Monday	Tuesday	Wednesday	Thursday	Friday	Saturday
Purpose	The Purpose of Sunday is To Reset and Refocus in a capacity WHICH WORKS FOR YOU	The Purpose Of Monday Is To SWITCH IT ON	The Purpose of Tuesday Is To STACK WINS	The Purpose of Wednesday Is To GENERATE MOMENTUM	The Purpose Of Thursday Is to TRY SOMETHING HARD	The Purpose Of Friday Is To EARN IT FOR THE WEEKEND	The Purpose Of Saturday Is To DO SOMETHING FUN OR NEW
Cardiovascular Endurance	Finish *Born to Run* by Christopher McDougall	3-Mile Run at 90% Heart Rate (180 bpm)	20-Minute Recovery Run Heart Rate at (160 bpm)	20 Minutes Low-impact Cardio (bike/ row/walk) Heart Rate at 110-120 bpm	20 Minutes Low-impact Cardio (bike/ row/walk) Heart Rate at 110-120 bpm	12-Mile Ruck For Time 35 lbs. Without Water Field Uniform and Boots	5 Minutes Low-impact Cardio (bike/row/walk) Heart Rate at 110- 120 bpm
Strength (unless specified) • **6 Sets x 3 Reps at a weight you can complete all 6 sets with**	Download and Listen to 1 interesting audio on either iTunes or Soundcloud by Fitness Podcast of Choice	Bench Press 3 Sets at 90% New 1RM	Back Squat 3 Sets at 90% New 1RM	None	None		None

"The Whole Man Program" WEEK 12 (Medium-Intensity and 12-Mile Ruck Test)

"The Whole Man Program" WEEK 12 (Medium-Intensity and 12-Mile Ruck Test)	Sunday	Monday	Tuesday	Wednesday	Thursday	Friday	Saturday
Muscular Endurance (unless specified) • **3 Exercises per muscle group** • **3-4 Sets x 15-20 Reps for Each Exercise** • **30 seconds to 1 minute rest between sets** • **2-3 minutes rest between exercises**	Discover and Research Athlete of Choice (use any platform available, Instagram, Snapchat, or the internet) Learn something new about weightlifting	Start With 2-3 Sets Medicine Ball Push-ups: 10 Wide, 10 Diamond, 10 Regular 30 Second Rest Between Sets —Then Do—Chest and Triceps Exercises for 20 Minutes. Do 3 Chest Exercises then 3 Triceps Exercises	3 Rounds for Time: 10 Body Weight Squat; 10 Body Weight Lunges (each leg); 10 Body Weight Sissy Squat; 10 V-ups	None	None	12-Mile Ruck For Time 35 lbs. Without Water Field Uniform and Boots	Sauna in Place of Lifting
Core For each Ab exercise you choose do 3 sets to failure, rest 30 seconds between sets and 2 minutes between exercises	None	None	None	None	None		None

"The Whole Man Program" WEEK 12 (Medium-Intensity and 12-Mile Ruck Test)

	Sunday	Monday	Tuesday	Wednesday	Thursday	Friday	Saturday
Mobility	None	Static Stretching	Foam Roll	Foam Roll and Stretch For 30 Minutes	Foam Roll and Stretch For 30 Minutes	Static Stretching	Foam Roll and Stretch For 30 Minutes
Goal	Self-Education	Taper	Taper	12-Mile Ruck Preparation	12-Mile Ruck Preparation	Personal Best on 12-Mile Ruck	Warm Up the Fascia and Muscles for Mobility, Flush out Toxins, Recover
Instructions	*Unlocking your Success Code* by Ed Mylett	*Born to Run* Review	Sissy Squats	How to Treat Cramps While Rucking	Foot Care, Blister Treatment	What to Focus on While Rucking, Immediately Treating Injuries and Agitations	None
Other	Visualization – Visualize Your Future Body, You Achieving Your Goals in Body, Mind, and Spirit. Visualize Perfect Balance and Discipline (10 Minutes)	**Meditate for 10 Minutes a day**	**Meditate for 10 Minutes**	**Meditate for 10 Minutes**	**Meditate for 10 Minutes**	**Meditate for 10 Minutes**	**Optional –Practice Visualization**

"Dominate LIFE"

Lesson for the Week: SUCCESS

B.O.D.Y. PROGRAMMING

I n order to ensure continued growth past the use of this program, I want to give you a tool I use to write my own programs. I use the acronym B.O.D.Y. to identify my workout goals and plug them into my training calendar. The result from going through B.O.D.Y. gives me the structure I need for a given week. From there, I allocate an intensity level and cycle the training. I typically use two high-intensity weeks followed by a medium- or low-intensity week. You can review this training program to see how I nested it in the progression we accomplished over the last 12 weeks. Here is the breakdown for B.O.D.Y. programming:

B – *Brainstorm* **your goals.** Grab a blank sheet of paper and write Professional and Personal at the top. Brainstorm all of the goals you have that fall into your fitness personal life and professional life. Spend 5-10 minutes brainstorming until you cannot think of any more goals. Consider both short- and long-term objectives. Select the goals you want to accomplish in the short term for the program you are going to write.

O – *Outline* **your workout split.** On a separate sheet of paper or calendar, fill in what days of the week you are going to dedicate to running, lifting, or the sport you are training for. This is your new workout split. Once you have completed the workout split, you should have the framework for your routine and have a timeline to achieve your goals. I like to write my programs four weeks at a time and make adjustments during the fifth week.

D – *Determine* your lifts. Write out what lifts you are going to need to do to accomplish your goals. Include running intervals. Plug these lifts into your workout split. For example, if Monday is chest and triceps, and you determined bench press as a goal, then you will do bench press on Monday to tackle that goal.

Y – Know your *why*. This is probably the most important step of programming. Most people have superficial goals that result in no accomplishments. You need to know WHY you want to accomplish each goal you listed. In order to discover that, pick one goal and write out all the ways you will feel if you are successful. Write out how you would feel if you do not reach it. Use single words to summarize the feeling. For example, use words like "respected" or "accomplished" or "confident." Do the same for the way you will feel if you do not accomplish each goal. Words like "disappointed" or "pathetic" are examples of strong negative feelings associated with failure. The feelings you write should feel powerful. If they are not, you need to reevaluate the goal. For example, if the idea of benching 315 lbs. makes you feel powerful and respected, it is a good goal. Determine your WHY for all of your goals and remind yourself of your why daily. Enjoy the journey.

SAMPLE TRAINING LOG

"The Whole Man" Programming Log

	Sunday	Monday	Tuesday	Wednesday	Thursday	Friday	Saturday
Purpose							
Cardiovascular Endurance							
Strength							
Muscular Endurance							

Core	Mobility	Goal	Mindset	Other	Your Motto for LIFE :-

NOTABLE QUOTES

"Life is long if you know how to life it." ~ Seneca

"Vague beginnings cause chaotic endings." ~ Jeramiah Solven

"The journey of a thousand miles begins with a single step." ~ Lao Tzu

"Insanity is doing the same thing over and over, but expecting a different result." ~ Albert Einstein

"The world is not a crazy enough of a place to reward a bunch of undeserving people." ~ Charlie Munger

"Perfection is not attainable, but if we chase it, we can achieve excellence." ~ Vince Lombardi

"It isn't what we say that defines us, it is what we do." ~ Jane Austen

"There is no change without a change in routine." ~ Tai Lopez

"Set the set piece before you move the move piece." ~ Military Philosophy

"An idle mind is the devil's playground, unless you master the playground." ~ Jeramiah Solven

"You cannot make more time but you can make better use of it." ~ Unknown

"Discipline equals freedom." ~ Jocko Willink

"Your focus determines your reality." ~ George Lucas

"Collect the dots and then connect the dots." ~ Pete Blaber

"Deliberate practice is purposeful, whereas practice is meaningless." ~ Jeramiah Solven

"Treat yourself do not cheat yourself" ~ Jeramiah Solven

"The chains of habit are too light to be felt until they are too heavy to be broken." ~ Warren Buffett

"A man who chases two rabbits catches none" ~ Chinese Proverb

"You cannot solve today's problems with yesterday's thinking." ~ Einstein

"Success in an inside job." ~ James Allen

"Do not get stuck sharpening your pencils." ~ Pete Drucker

"Do not put off tomorrow, what you can do today." ~ Ben Franklin

"The man who thinks he can and the man who thinks he cannot are both right." ~ Chinese Proverb

"A nation is born stoic and dies epicurean." ~ Will Duran

"Judge a man not by what he has achieved but by who is at his funeral." ~ Jeramiah Solven

"Life happens for us not to us." ~ Anthony Robbins

"You can lead a horse to water but you cannot make him drink." ~ John Heywood

"Busyness is a sign of laziness." ~ Tim Ferris

"Infuse heart, soul, spirit, and passion because talent is not enough." ~ Dominick Cruz

RULES TO LIVE BY

Be 1% better every day.

Practice breaking through failure.

Learn to be comfortable being uncomfortable.

Make a habit of choosing the harder option.

Seek inches not miles.

Develop a system for personal growth.

Exercise self-care routinely in a capacity that works for you.

Constantly seek out opportunities that challenge you.

Give more than you receive but receive well.

Help everyone you can to achieve success but do not drag them there.

Bring out the best in people.

Be appreciative for even the smallest of things.

Be relentless in your pursuit of your best self.

Allow your passion to steer you through life.

Consistently recognize you only live once and make decisions that maximize your experience.

~ Jeramiah Solven

CONTACT INFORMATION

If you enjoyed the book and want to stay connected, follow me on Instagram @jeramiahsolven. For questions, comments, or additional training, direct message me or contact me by email at info@jeramiahsolven.com.

#DOMINATELIFE

PODCASTS AND THOUGHT LEADERS

Andy Frisella (@andyfrisella) – *The MFCEO Project*

Annie Dohack (@anniegunshow) – *Iron and Lead Podcast*

BedrosKeuilian (@bedroskeuilian) – *Empire Podcast Show*

Chris Patterson (@chrispatterson) – *livelargecoaching.com*

David Meltzer (@davidmeltzer) – *The Playbook*

Ed Mylett (@edmylett) – *Ed Mylett Show*

Jocko Willink (@jockowillink) – *Jocko Podcast*

Joe Rogan (@joerogan) – *The Joe Rogan Show*

Lewis Howes (@lewishowes) – *The School of Greatness*

Shawn Stevenson (@shawnmodel) – *The Model Health Show*

Tai Lopez (@tailopez) – *The Tai Lopez Show*

Tim Ferris (@timferris) – *The Tim Ferris Show*

BOOKS

30 Minute Expert Summaries. *Summary - the Power of Habit ... in 30 Minutes: A Concise Summary of Charles Duhigg's Bestselling Book*. 30 Minute Expert Summaries Series. Berkeley, CA: Garamond Press, 2012.

Breus, Michael, and Mehmet Oz. *The Power of When: Discover Your Chronotype--and the Best Time to Eat Lunch, Ask for a Raise, Have Sex, Write a Novel, Take Your Meds, and More*. New York: Little, Brown Spark, 2019.

Centrella, Sarah. *Hustle Believe Receive: An 8-step Plan to Changing Your Life and Living Your Dream*. Read by Marisa Vitali. Newark: Audible, 2016.

Collins, Jim. *Good to Great: Why Some Companies Make the Leap and Others Don't*. New York: HarperBusiness, 2001.

Ferriss, Timothy. *The 4-hour Work Week: Escape the 9-5, Live Anywhere and Join the New Rich*. London: Vermillion, 2008.

Frankl, Viktor E., and Alexander Batthyany. *The Feeling of Meaninglessness - a Challenge to Psychotherapy and Philosophy*. Marquette University Press, 2010.

Gladwell, Malcolm. *Outliers: The Story of Success*. New York: Back Bay Books, Little, Brown and Company, 2019.

Lee, Kibeom, and Michael Craig Ashton. *The H Factor of Personality: Why Some People Are Manipulative, Self-Entitled, Materialistic, and Exploitive - and Why It Matters for Everyone*. Ontario: Wilfrid Laurier University Press, 2013.

Lee, Kibeom, and Michael Craig Ashton. *The HEXACO Personality Inventory-Revised*. Retrieved October 5, 2018, from http://hexaco.org/

Losier, Michael J. *Law of Attraction: The Science of Attracting More of What You Want and Less of What You Don't*. New York: Grand Central Publishing, 2019.

McChrystal, Stanley A., Tantum Collins, David Silverman, and Chris Fussell. *Team of Teams: New Rules of Engagement for a Complex World*. New York: Portfolio/Penguin, 2015.

Robbins, Mel. *The 5 Second Rule: The Fastest Way to Change Your Life*. Nashville, TN: Savio Republic, 2017.

www.ingramcontent.com/pod-product-compliance
Lightning Source LLC
Chambersburg PA
CBHW070758270326
41927CB00010B/2200